BECOMING
DOCTORS
25 Years Later

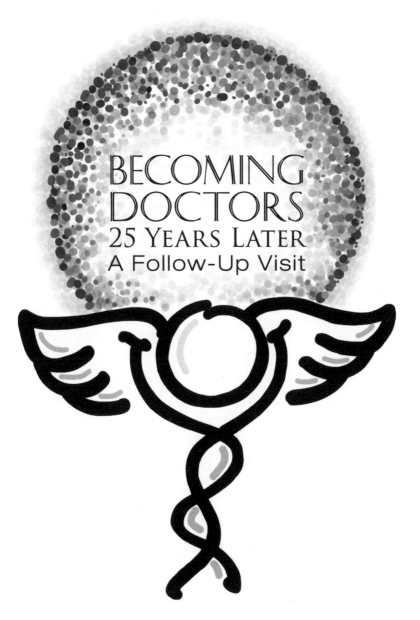

BECOMING DOCTORS
25 YEARS LATER
A Follow-Up Visit

EDITED BY PAR BOLINA M.D.

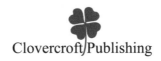

Clovercroft Publishing

Becoming Doctors 25 Years Later

©2021 by Par Bolina

Published by Clovercroft Publishing, Franklin, Tennessee.

www.clovercroftpublishing.com

Cover illustration by Dr. Sue Rhee

Cover Design by Adept Concept Solutions

Interior Design by Adept Content Solutions

ISBN: 978-1-950892-98-3

Printed in the United States of America

CONTENTS

PREFACE

After enjoying extraordinary prosperity for over half a century, humanity is collectively experiencing the first "world war" of the twenty-first century. One that is challenging the global population, its clinical soldiers and scientists, and our way of life. The pandemic of 2020 serves as a humbling reminder of our limitations and vulnerabilities as we mount a response to the crisis.

Fortunately, the investment placed in science, technology, and medicine by generations before us has enabled us to rapidly develop vaccinations and treatments that may avert global catastrophe. If this crisis passes with limited death and destruction, our commitment to science and knowledge, peace and collaboration, and openness and transparency will perhaps be deeper and broader than ever before. Over centuries and millennia, such victories of human ingenuity add to the compelling body of evidence supporting diversity of thought and equality in opportunity as key contributors to innovation and prosperity for all.

Now, in an unusual sequel anthology, we present a more personal example of diversity of thought and equality of opportunity as reflected in the journey of twenty-five physicians. We first met them twenty-five years ago when they shared their stories and experiences of being medical students in the book *Becoming* Doctors. After studying at Brown, Cornell, Emory, Johns Hopkins, Stanford, Yale, and a dozen more medical schools, these doctors went on to become emergency medicine physicians, family practitioners, gynecologists, internists, obstetricians, pediatricians, psychiatrists, and surgeons across the United States. Today, while working alongside the clinical soldiers and scientists protecting our friends and neighbors from this pandemic, they share their personal insights of learning, practicing, and teaching medicine over the past twenty-five years. Their essays, stories, drawings, and poems form this unique anthology, capturing their aspirations and struggles as students and their challenges and successes as physicians, parents, and teachers.

Over the last three decades since they decided to become doctors, these physicians tell us of the gratification, joy, and fulfillment of their work coupled with their experiences of uncertainty, fear, and disappointment. They share how their professional responsibilities impact their personal lives while caring for their patients and how living up to the expectations of their colleagues and community often conflicts with the needs of their family.

Through their words, we hear the personal toll becoming a doctor has taken. Yet, regardless of diversity in gender, faith, or race, these doctors embrace healing even when they may be suffering, teaching even as they continue their learning and reassuring even as they seek better methods, ideas, and solutions. Not surprisingly, when asked whether they would make the same career choice or whether they would recommend a career in medicine for their children, they reaffirm the decision to become doctors. Perhaps such predictability is best explained by an innovative thinker and gracious teacher from the past century, Albert Einstein, who said, "Only a life lived for others is a life worthwhile." Given the opportunity, these physicians have done just that.

Par Bolina, M.D.
Editor

CLINIC

Ten weeks down in my surgery clerkship, two to go. I am so beat, so exhausted that I can't even walk fast anymore. Traversing the parking lot on the way into the hospital today seemed like crossing the steppe, and I staggered twice as I labored to reach my once-a-week primary care clinic. Normally, anything that gets me away from the drudgery of the OR is anticipated, but by now, I am so whipped that just arriving at clinic is a monumental effort. The depths of my fatigue have reached the point where I am too tired to complain. I stare blankly at friends who wish me well in the elevator, trying to place them. I fall asleep at home with the lights blazing and the doors unlocked. If we get an admission after four, I want to cry, but I can't muster up the energy.

"Here she is, our little bundle of joy," one of the residents says as I shuffle into the conference room. The medical interns are tired too, but largely happy—drinking gourmet coffee out of paper cups from the hospital's upscale croissant joint, crossing off the day's tasks on their lists, and conferring by phone with the specialists who are seeing their patients in consultation. They have interesting jobs; they don't have to stand stock-still for six hours at a time hauling on a slippery retractor and trying to recall how many days ago their last meal was. After I plop into one of the straight-backed chairs at the conference table, they go on telling the story they had started about a patient in the unit who developed ICU psychosis and got as far as the automatic doors but couldn't figure out how to open them by pressing the plate on the wall. "It was change of shift," the second year says. "All the nurses were eating coffee cake in the lounge. It was the maintenance man who noticed he was flying the coop." They all laugh—young, vital people in their twenties who have chosen to postpone the rest of their lives so they can prevent crazy nutcakes from leaving the unit at midnight.

"Your first patient is here," one of the medical assistants tells me, tossing the chart on the table in front of me. It is large and very thick, a patient I haven't seen before. It figures. I was kind of hoping everyone would just cancel today. I consider opening the chart and trying to read about this person who is waiting for me, but the task seems too monumental. "Oh." I can't even come up with an expletive good enough to convey my state of mind. "God," I wind up sighing.

My patient is a very skinny black man in sunglasses and a wheelchair pushed by his sister. I instantly regret not reading the chart. There is something very wrong with this guy—tertiary syphilis, maybe. He's twitching like crazy. I try to shake his hand, then wind up directing most of my greeting at the sister, who looks at me as if I were the last human being on earth after the Holocaust. This is going to be good. I'm going to have to sit down for this one. I realize, dimly, that I was so tired after slugging across the parking lot that I forgot to eat lunch. That makes breakfast yesterday my last meal.

"It's really nice to meet you," I tell the sister. "You guys have been coming here for a long time." I heft the chart in my hand so she knows whence I speak. "But I haven't met you myself, so I need to ask you just some basic things about your brother's medical history."

"He has some disease," she says anxiously. "I don't know what it's called, but he ain't going to get better, that's what they told us. It runs in the family or something."

I flip through the chart until I find the neatly typed, dictated neurology notes. "Forty-year-old male with Huntington's disease," one of them begins. Huntington's. These facts permeate my sleepy brain as I look more closely at the man, his arms twitching aimlessly in an asynchronous dance. The autosomal dominant chorea that we all memorized as first-year students in genetics class. Woody Guthrie. It comes back to me in a rush. I would have paid good money back then to see a real, live patient with advanced Huntington's. I would have thought it fascinating. Now here he is, a living exercise in physical diagnosis, and it is all unbearably sad.

"How has he been doing lately?" I ask softly, focusing better on the sister. The patient has made no move toward me, given no indication that he understands. I will speak instead to her, reassure her, and if he hears us, he will know we care.

"Bad," she says, tears rising up in her eyes. "That's why we came. I can't take care of him no more. I just can't do it. I try, oh, God, I try, but lately . . ." She shakes her head. He can no longer walk, dress himself, or feed himself. He is incontinent. He goes into rages and strikes her—once knocking her against the bathroom mirror. She has small grandchildren at home whom she also has to care for. She doesn't know what to do now, but she has brought him here to me today in hopes that I can work a miracle.

"He's lucky to have you," I tell her reassuringly. "It sounds like you've done a great job taking care of him at home for as long as you could, but no one expects you to have to keep this up forever. What I can do is try to make arrangements for a nursing home, and in the meantime get a visiting nurse to come by and help you out at home."

"I know he probably doesn't want to go to a nursing home," she says guiltily, clenching her hands together in her lap.

"No one likes the idea," I say, "but they would know how best to take care of him there. They're very good at it, and you'd visit him often, I know."

"Oh, every day," she says. "Oh, doctor, I feel bad."

"I understand," I say, taking her hand. "You've done a great job taking care of him this long at home. I know he appreciates it, even if he gets confused sometimes."

"Where's he going to go?" she wants to know.

"I need to make some calls," I say. "Okay? Then I'll come back, and we can talk about things in more detail. Can you guys hang on a few minutes?"

"We've been hanging on all these weeks; a few more minutes is okay," she says tremulously, grasping her brother's hand and bringing it up to her mouth to kiss it.

In the conference room, I am guided through the maze of paperwork one needs to make a referral to an "extended care facility." One of the questions is whether the patient is expected to live longer than six months. I write, "No," and then look at it for a long time. If I write it, will it happen? Am I wishing an early death on him? But what would be better, really, at this point? Best that he should code today, in clinic, before things get really bad. I am reminded, in these philosophic riddles, that he needs a code status, preferably before the nursing home. God forbid this poor guy gets intubated by some overzealous resident in the ER who sees his age and goes for the big save the night he finally stops breathing.

Mary, the nurse on my team, gets on the phone to several area nursing homes. She is a wide-eyed, efficient person who chews gum like it's going out of style. "Barbara," she says in a familiar way to the second place.

"Mary. Got any beds for a forty-year-old guy with—what does he have? Huntington's disease? I don't know, it's like a progressive neuro thing. Yeah, he's gonna die. Wheelchair bound, incontinent . . . yeah. Well, the thing is, they just can't care for him anymore. . . . Okay, I'll make you a deal. I'll wash your car if you can get him in by next Saturday. Well, when do you think she's going to die? Well, how about we make him next available bed then? . . . It'll have to be." She cuts her eyes to me. I'm nodding enthusiastically. "Okay with the doctor. She's doing them now. Good. Here's their number." She reads it off from the front page of the chart. "Any meds?" she asks me.

"I'm going to start him on some Haldol," I say. "For agitation." "Just Haldol," she says into the receiver. "Yeah, Barb, thanks." "You're washing her car?" I say in disbelief when she hangs up.

"Whatever it takes," Mary says with a shrug.

The sister is weeping. I have just explained the nursing home situation to her, and she cries in guilt and relief and exhaustion. "I'll get you some help over the next week or so, until they're ready for him," I say, rubbing my eyes. "Now there's a few other things I need to talk to you about. Does your brother have any kids?"

"Two," she says. "He never sees them."

"Well, here's the thing. This disease he has runs in families. So, his kids have a fifty-fifty chance that they could develop it too. There's a test that they can take, if they want, to detect it early. How old are they?"

"Eighteen and fifteen," she says after calculating a moment. "Well, they have time to decide," I say. "But maybe you could have them come in and see me. We can talk about it together. How about you guys? Did you and your other brother ever get tested?"

"No," she says.

"And how old are you now?"

"Forty-nine," she says. "My brother's forty-six."

"Okay," I tell her. "This disease usually comes on in the thirties, or early forties, so I'd say it's less likely that you'll get it. But if you want to get tested. . . ."

"I'll talk to my brother about it."

"Fine. You can call me if you have any questions about that part of it," I say. "The other thing I wanted to bring up with you was how much you want done for your brother if he gets real sick." I rest my hand on his knee as I say this in case he can hear. "I don't think that's going to happen soon, but I also don't think he has a real long time to go. And because he's young, you know, people will be very willing to say, okay, let's do everything, and they may not know how sick he really is . . ."

She considers this. "Oh, we don't want him to be kept alive, you know, a vegetable or anything like that," she says tentatively.

"So, like, if he were to stop breathing, or his heart stopped, you wouldn't want them to try to bring him back? Or bring him to the hospital?"

"Um . . . I guess not," she says softly. "I feel real bad about this. I wish he could tell me what to do."

"Well, you can try to think about the kinds of things he would have wanted back when he was still talking to you," I say. "You know your brother better than anybody, so you're really the best person to make that decision."

She looks back at me anxiously.

"Okay," I say, taking charge. "So, you don't want them to do anything heroic, like putting a tube down his throat if he stops breathing, or trying to keep him alive past the point where he's really . . ."

"Exactly," she says, relieved to have this conversation over with.

"I think that's good," I tell her.

"You do?"

"Yes." I would say this regardless of her choice, of course, but I really do happen to agree with her, so it's easier. "We'll make sure that the people in the nursing home know that too, so everyone's in agreement. Okay?"

"Okay," she says.

We meet at the desk in the waiting room on their way out so I can give her the Haldol prescription and the phone numbers for VNA and the nursing home. It is almost four. I notice, somewhere from the fog that has permeated my brain, that my other two patients for today didn't show. A very good thing too, as all I want right now is to go into the conference room and put my head down on the table and sleep for about sixteen hours.

My patient conducts invisible symphonies from his chair as his sister watches him in undeniable sorrow. When I hand her the nursing home papers, she begins to sob, and I think for a moment that her guilt at having to place him there will overcome her. Then I realize they are tears of relief. When she hugs me, in a sudden impulsive goodbye, she all but squeezes the life out of me. "Doctor, I can never thank you enough for this day," she whispers.

I get my knapsack from the conference room and check twice to make sure I have my keys—they have a surprising habit of disappearing when

I am post-call. As I leave, the secretaries all tell me how bad I look, something they've adopted during my surgery rotation. They give advice on what I should do to feel better—hot bath, square meal, sleep, or a massage. At this point, remaining upright until I get to my car sounds like a challenge enough.

Downstairs, I veer into the coffee shop before I go, deciding that a bagel is a good idea. If I can find the change in my pockets. If I can find my pockets. In the mirrored window behind the cashier, I catch a glimpse of the doctor my patient saw, the one who found a nursing home for her brother. I realize that when he dies, it will be this day she remembers most, the day his death became a reality for her. The memory of the doctor who helped her decide will stay with her till the day she dies. Today, I have been in the eye of someone else's hurricane.

I pay for my bagel and start to eat it slowly as I put one blood-spattered clog in front of the other on my way out the door.

Joanne Wilkinson
Brown University School of Medicine
Class of 1995

DINNERTIME

I've been out of med school for twenty-five years now. Somehow, I thought by now I would be the beloved owner of my own practice, my name on the lips of every family in town . . . or a full professor sitting comfortably in my booklined office . . . and in between I would rush in and out of the hospital, my white coat starched and clean, to provide impressive and timely medical care without messing up my hair.

Instead, this happens: It's a Tuesday night. I'm on service. I have eight patients, and I saw seven of them this morning (no white coat and no starch, just gray wrapover black pants and clogs). The eighth was off the floor for a test, and I tried again at lunch, but then she was in endoscopy, so I left to pick up my daughter from school. When we got home, she was upset about failing her math test, so I had to sit with her on the couch for a little while and go through the test with her to figure out what went wrong. Then I looked up and the sun was falling in the sky. It was almost five, and I still hadn't seen my last patient. I asked my kid if she was okay staying home by herself for forty minutes while I ran over to the hospital, but she wasn't. So I bundled her into the car and took her with me.

Now it's 5:20. The hospital lobby is streaming with visitors. I have fallen even below the black pants and gray unstructured wrap standard and am now wearing black pants and a gray fleece sweatshirt that is warm but not new. It doesn't make me look like a doctor. Also, my hair is kind of straggly. Also, my ten-year-old is bopping along next to me, hoping I will lose my head and take her shopping in the gift shop. I promised her a dinner out at the trendy pizza place when we were done here. I park her on a chair in the lobby near a bunch of sedate-looking women in their seventies. (When I come back, she will tell me that they left almost immediately, to be replaced by a "guy in a hoodie who got thrown out by the security guards," for what

I don't know. I will respond, mildly, that I have a hoodie too.) I walk as fast as I can back to the endoscopy unit, hoping that my patient isn't so zonked after her EGD that she doesn't remember me coming to see her.

The unit is dark except for one patient: my lady, frail and over ninety, but alert and sharp as a tack after two of Versed and twenty-five of Fentanyl. The nurses in this unit don't know me and think I am her daughter coming to visit. I point, wordlessly, at my badge. (In case you are wondering, over the last twenty-five years, I have reminded people that I am, in fact, the doctor, on average five times per day.) "You survived," I say succinctly to my patient, who takes my hand in her own frail, skeletal one.

"I guess I did," she says, as though surprised herself. She has been losing weight, and while I think it's depression, we needed to make sure her EGD was normal. She asks where my daughter is. Why was I coming to see her so late in the day? She wants to make sure I have something planned for my daughter's dinner. When I name the restaurant we are planning to visit, she relaxes. Ever the caretaker, she worries about my ten-year-old getting enough to eat while in the midst of her own medical workup near the end of her life.

I don't have a mother—or a grandmother—who calls me and worries about these things. My patients are my family, for better or worse. I have arrived at this midlife place without many supports—my dad is nearby; I have a best friend who is battling cancer and busy with her own family; I have neighbors who take in my trash cans while I'm at work. That's it. My daughter's friends' parents are nice and helpful when I ask for it, but there is no one who calls me up on Saturday mornings and asks me if I need a bagel delivery or offers to babysit. Not even anyone who worries that my sweet pea won't eat enough on a school night. My patients, bless them, do this.

I squeeze my patient's hand. I tell her that so far, everything looks normal and we think she needs to go home to be with her family and eat chicken soup. And McDonald's. And ice cream when she is in the mood. She weighs barely one hundred pounds, about ten pounds more than the gourmet pizza eater who awaits me in the lounge. "I am coming to see you at home next week, and I want to see empty takeout containers all over the house," I tell her in my most threatening way. She squeezes back and laughs. "Take good care of your girl," she tells me. "I always do," I say back.

It's strange how the years pass. When I was younger, I had a simpler view of my life: I would attain certain milestones because I deserved them, not too early and not too late; I would proceed majestically through my career, through dating and marriage and having children, and arrive at retirement with a full complement of adoring fans. I didn't anticipate job changes, lateral moves, and eating crackers alone in front of my laptop at dinnertime. I didn't anticipate that my patients would become my family. I didn't anticipate that the caring and the work would flow both ways.

My patient looks me in the eye. "I'm good," she says. "Go take your daughter for pizza." She gives my hand one last squeeze, and then she lets me go.

Joanne Wilkinson, M.D.
Family Medicine

PERSONAL STATEMENT

Two dreams. One will go unfilled for lack of great talent. The other will be realized and become my life's devotion. Two different dreams that share much in common.

Two players. Both don uniforms. One is pinstriped and includes cleats. The other is green and includes shoe covers. Both uniforms appear to disguise the individual personalities from casual observers. Yet, each player may excel in his respective profession.

Two arenas. Both players are rookies. The first struggled through the minor league, where he was coached by professionals about the intricacies of baseball. The second endured years of schooling and residency to train for the art of surgery. Neither player ever stops learning about his respective game.

The new pitcher controls the flow of the game on the field. He shakes off the sign from the catcher because he knows a different pitch will be more effective. The pitcher has the ability to strike out the side or to toss the pitch that will be the game-ending home run. His teammates, as well as the fans, place their trust in him. The new surgeon controls the flow of the game in the operating room. The nurses, the anesthesiologist, and the assistants all play vital parts in the game but must take their cues from the surgeon. As the pitcher calls for a pitch, the surgeon delivers the instrument to the patient. The pitch and the instrument called for were wise decisions made by skilled professionals. The pitcher saved the game for his team and his fans. The surgeon saved a life for the patient and the patient's family and friends.

Only recently have I realized a major difference between these two players—commitment. It has been said that there are two types of creatures on the face of the earth: those with a commitment and those who require

10

the commitment of others. Physicians possess a commitment unique in scope and importance. From the moment an ill or injured person enters the office or emergency department, a relationship develops between physician and patient. This relationship is so deeply rooted in the tenets of compassion, honesty, and trust that it cannot be rivaled by a mere pitcher and his catcher.

Surgery, unlike baseball, is commitment. It is the commitment to ensure that your patient receives the best care possible. It is the commitment to endless days, sleepless nights, and tasteless cafeteria food. It is the commitment to celebrate with a family's happiness and to grieve with their losses. It is the commitment to a new education with each new patient. It is the commitment to do it all again the next day.

Two players. Of the first it is said that as long as the pitcher can keep the ball off the fat part of the bat, the sweet spot, then he is doing his job. Of the second, it is said that you will never trust anyone in your life the way you trust your surgeon.

Two dreams. One will fade into a weekend hobby. The other will be realized and become my life's devotion.

Keith D. Mortman
University of Medicine and Dentistry of New Jersey
Robert Wood Johnson Medical School
Class of 1994

TWENTY-FIVE
YEARS

Twenty-five years since medical school. It has been a dizzying career that has taken me across the country and back again. Much has transpired since the first pitch of my surgical training. Much has been learned since my rookie days. Many have been saved. A few have been lost. They have all taught me something about the game of medicine, surgery, life, or myself.

Twenty-five years of rising before dawn and donning my uniform of scrubs and shoe covers. I arrive at the ballpark before a crow has had its first cup of coffee. Today will be a good day because I will continue to practice my craft alongside the other dedicated members of my team. Time has reinforced the belief that surgery is the epitome of team sports. Though I am seen as the captain, the team cannot take the field without the surgical assistant, the anesthesiologist, the scrub technician, the circulating nurse, the pathologist, the oncologist, and the radiologist. And the game cannot be played without the respiratory therapist, the lab technician, the intensivist, the patient transporter, the unit clerk, and the cafeteria worker. Each plays a vital role and contributes to the team. Appreciate them. Thank them.

Twenty-five years of learning. The pitcher does not stop perfecting his slider once drafted into the major leagues. The pitching coach is responsible for developing the neophyte into a seasoned veteran. There are countless hours of practice with the catcher in the bullpen or at the park, sometimes in the rain and often as the day's light fades. So too does the surgeon continue to learn. Each patient tells a new story that I add to my growing book of knowledge, skill, and judgment. To be a surgeon is to have a thirst for this knowledge and the desire to continually discover. Today I am not a senior attending surgeon—I am a PGY 25, a professional student.

Twenty-five years has brought me two wives, three children, three dogs, seven states, and thirteen homes. The game of surgery can be an arduous one. It is said that one should cherish their children while they are young because though the days are long, the years are short. The days of surgery are just as long. Surgery, like baseball, respects no clock. The game is nine innings, no matter how long it takes. Sometimes it lasts two hours. Sometimes it is twelve hours and stretches past the setting sun, two meals, three bathroom breaks, and multiple operating room shift changes. Success here is not measured by keeping the ball off the fat part of the bat or keeping runs off the scoreboard. Success in the operating room is defined by complete resection of the tumor with negative margins, a perfect anastomosis that does not leak blood or enteric contents, or reconstruction of the chest wall and diaphragm to allow normal respiration.

Twenty-five years has taught me that success in the operating room is really defined by a smooth emergence from anesthesia. By having the patient wake up at the end of the operation. By having the patient sail through the hospitalization without complication. By the tears of gratitude from the patient's spouse or child after telling them of a successful surgical outcome. By the holiday cards and pictures that I receive from patients documenting another year of being cancer-free. By the calls from colleagues asking my expert opinion about a complex case. By performing research and having my findings accepted by a prestigious journal or presented at an international meeting. By the privilege of mentoring dozens, teaching hundreds, and caring for thousands over twenty-five years.

Twenty-five years. As I enter the later innings of my surgical career, I look back on my medical student self. He was young and naïve certainly. Yet he was not too far off the mark. Commitment is, in fact, at the core of the surgeon's practice. Some days do seem endless. Some nights are sleepless. Sometimes the cafeteria food is tasteless. But every patient and every day brings with it a commitment for a new education. A commitment to do it all over again the next day.

Twenty-five years. Though I approach the later innings of the game, it's a beautiful day for a doubleheader. Let's do it again.

Keith D. Mortman, M.D.
Thoracic Surgery

SCIENCE CAMP

Mother sent me to science camp the summer I turned ten,
Though I would rather have spent the days
Acting scared as Pat Barger dug nightcrawlers from under his porch,
Enough for more fish
Than any boy could hook in one summer.

But at camp, we searched through Illinois cornrows,
Looking for upturned pieces of flint
That could have been parts
Of arrowheads and Indian tools.
We hunted for geodes along forested creeks

More lovely than anything at 840 Elm Street.

She had sent me, hoping she'd keep me from dreaming
Of becoming a princess, a model,
A wife.
But she frowned at the end when Dad brought me back

With a cartful of rocks that would litter her flower patch,

And I asked her daily for a boa constrictor.

Gillian S. Herald
University of Illinois College of Medicine at Chicago
Class of 1997

MY YEAR WITH SUZANNE

"Bitch!" Suzanne calls after me. I have lost my clout. The staff, the other patients, and I are again her enemies. I should have known we would be in for a wild ride when I showed up this morning to the inpatient psychiatric unit and she greeted me with full manic makeup: bright blue eyeshadow, thick painted eyebrows, and cheeks and lips a bruised red. Over months of treatment trying to help her become competent to stand trial, she has gone from nonstop rage to a few weeks at a time of reasonable "bargaining" about her treatment, and now back to mania.

I work in one of the country's largest forensic state psychiatric hospitals. My patients are all women at some stage of involvement in the criminal justice system. Almost always, they arrive without an understanding of why they are sent here. Their crimes (or alleged crimes) are generally felonies, often violent, often influenced by psychosis—for example, delusional belief that someone is trying to hurt them and acting accordingly. A large part of mental illness is lack of awareness that one has it. Thus, most often, my patients are not receiving psychiatric treatment when these crimes occur. Their life circumstances have not been conducive to trusting others. They have been navigating a mental health system that is fragmented and underfunded. Patients who show up, if they are fortunate, can get treatment; those who don't are lost to care until they end up in jail or prison.

When I sit down with Suzanne a couple of months later, she has brought some pieces of candy into the meeting—her proceeds from her wins at Scrabble and Bingo. I comment that her current medications seem to be working and suggest no further changes, so she can finally leave the hospital and get back to court. She smiles, places two fingers on the Jolly Rancher, and slyly slides it my direction. "I will give you two of these if you take away a pill of Depakote," she tries. She knows that the next step is a court case, but she feels she has already done her time. She asks when she is going to be able to be totally free, so she can do the things she has planned for the future—get a driver's license, go back to college, and see her nieces and nephews. I don't have an answer.

Suzanne has spent most of the past twenty years in and out of hospitals, jails, prisons, and other institutions. Now she is eager to get back to court so she can tell her side of the story about the most recent charges. What that story turns out to be will be up to her and her lawyer and is not a concern in treatment. Our job is just to help her get there—to ensure that she understands the process and can be calm and safe in the courtroom. For months now, we have done this dance—she gets close to being ready, then she starts to refuse a critical medication, and her behavior again becomes unpredictable and dangerous.

But the day comes when I sit with Suzanne as she waits to leave with the hospital police for jail and her upcoming court date. The belongings she has packed fill just one paper bag—some makeup and nail polish, two books, a tube of hair product, and some candy and chips from the hospital canteen. As she walks off the unit, I wonder if Suzanne will be comfortable enough to try to bargain candy with her new psychiatric team. When she waivers in her opinion about needing the treatment, will she let them help her continue? I am reminded of the credo from my department chair a couple of decades ago when I was still in training: "Remember, psychiatry is fundamentally about the relationship."

Gillian Herald Friedman, M.D.
Psychiatry

GOING FOR THE JUGULAR

Mistakes will happen even at the best of medical schools. When the von Trapenbergs presented their newly departed family head to the anatomy lab at this particular school, no one suspected that the corpse was not a corpse at all, but rather, a snoozing vampire. The medical faculty simply were not trained in such matters. Thus, as often seems to occur, these scientists overlooked the obvious, heading smugly back to labs and offices when they should have been cowering in fear, or at least anxiously rounding up members for a new committee.

Otto von Trapenberg himself did not know how he'd ended up on an aluminum table, his body steeped in foul-smelling chemicals and wrapped in a plastic sheet. He suspected that his wife had had something to do with it. Otto had seen Betty sizing up the pizza boy the night before his ill-fated nap and flirting with the gas station attendant the evening before that on their way to see the grandkids in that infernal show, *The Sound of Music*. Damn whiskers on kittens! Screw warm woolen mittens! It wasn't his fault, Otto brooded, if he weren't up to old standards as far as pleasing his wife. After all, he was pushing three hundred years old.

Three hundred years and still struggling to get by. Could Otto retire, move south, and take up a life of golf and bingo? No sirree. A vampire's work was never done. Always lusting for blood, fleeing the sun, and trying to keep up a classy appearance in a world where satin-lined capes were increasingly hard to come by. And to make matters more difficult, Otto now had this new situation of playing cadaver so as not to startle the kids.

The embalming chemicals had kept Otto woozy for a few days after he awoke in the lab. By the time he'd returned to his senses, the kids had already stripped half the skin off his legs. Being a polite old bat, Otto could not leave them now, even though, as you can imagine, an anatomy lab was not the most pleasant place for a vampire to be. There were all those glaring lights in one's eyes, the nasty scalpels slitting one's skin, and the latex-sheathed hands yanking out fat and pulling back layers of muscle. Luckily, the nerves were pretty well pickled. Otto felt only the slightest shiver, say, when David ran his fingers along the length of a nerve in his arm, chanting, "Ulnar, ulnar, ulnar," to engrain the strange syllables into his feeble memory. Otto thought that he himself could fare better on any test than these students could, but then he'd always had a sharp mind. Sharp mind, sharp teeth, hot blood . . .

How agonizing, these three students crowded around one's bed, their fresh young blood sugar-laced with vending machine candy and their resistance low from long hours of hitting the books. David might be stupid, but he looked like a tasty one, and Stan was temptingly fat. Then there was Marianna . . . sweet Marianna. The boys often gave her a hard time, teasing because she was more squeamish than they and more easily exhausted. But that was only because Marianna had sensitivity, feelings. She performed her dissections with patience and respect, unlike the other dolts, who just hacked through to make their grades. Dear Marianna. How Otto would like to take a scalpel to *her* pliant flesh, to drain her blood with his parched and eager lips.

Several weeks into the semester came a perfect night for prowling. The moon was full, the lab was empty, and Otto was ravenous. He thrust off his wrappings and sat up on the table. A few loose pieces of skin fell to the floor. No biggie.

Otto leaped from the table, thrust out his wings, and slipped out the window, which the students kept open to ease the room's smell. Ah, freedom. Otto savored the feel of brisk night air on his fuzzy body as he flapped along to Marianna's place. Otto kept his ears perked during dissections, so he knew exactly how to find her neat white townhouse. The windows were closed, however, so Otto had to squeeze through the crack under the front door. Luckily, bats are fairly flat, so they can do that sort of squeezing.

Inside the apartment, Otto switched back to human form. Woops. He'd forgotten that he'd been naked. Otto dodged into the kitchen and found a half apron. It had a ruffle around the edge and a stenciled row of Scottie dogs. Now, Otto had always been a classy guy—high starched collars, cummerbunds, the works—even after most of his fellow undead had proclaimed such accoutrements passé. But in a pinch like this, the apron would do.

Tying the apron at his waist, Otto headed out of the kitchen, through the living room, and up a plushly carpeted flight of stairs. Loose skin and muscles flapped on his back as he walked. His legs felt unsteady and light since so much fat had been removed. Darling Marianna herself had stripped the pads of fat from the soles of his feet. The exposed nerves gave the slightest tingle each time they hit the floor.

At the top of the stairs was a door with a slit of light beneath. Otto pushed it open, and there was Marianna asleep at her desk. Her head rested on an arm, which leaned on an anatomy atlas that lay open to a cutaway view of an armpit. *She must have been thinking of me as she drifted to sleep*, Otto mused. He had always been a romantic.

Otto stepped closer, noting the tendrils of hair curling around Marianna's face, the curve of her shoulders, and an empty carton of rocky road ice cream at the side of the desk. Her blood would taste of chocolate. Otto's stomach gurgled in anticipation. Marianna's head jerked. She spun around.

"Uncle Sam!" Marianna cried. Otto winced. He hated that nickname, invented by Stan. The nincompoop had mistaken his tattoo of the phoenix, symbol of immortality, for a bald eagle getting its feathers singed off by a cherry bomb. The tattoo had been Otto's gift to himself on his 275th birthday. Betty had said he'd regret it. "Just you wait and see if I'm right," Betty had shrieked many times. But here was Marianna, considerate and kind. The kind of girl who would never say, "I told you so."

Otto swept Marianna's hair to the side of her neck.

"Sam!" the girl cried, grabbing his hand. She looked pleadingly into his eyes. "Be a doll, Uncle Sam, and let me see your underarm for a minute. I'm still not straight on the brachial plexus."

Otto raised his arm and let Marianna pick through the tangle of nerves.

"Ah, *there's* the musculocutaneous," she finally sighed. Marianna turned to verify the finding in her book. Otto seized the moment to plunge forward to her neck, so white and sweet; his teeth slid in deep, and the blood frothed in his mouth like an ice cream soda. Otto tasted those marshmallow swirls. Delicious.

The next thing Otto knew, he was back in the lab. David was examining his neck while Stan stood nearby, tearing open a pack of M&M's.

"I guess this is the sternothyroid muscle, so this would be the sterno-hyoid," David was saying. The words throbbed in Otto's ears. The table seemed to spin, first in one direction and then the other. Otto felt ancient. He never used to get hangovers. He had never blacked out before. He had never lain in bed the next morning like this, unable to recall how he'd returned. Otto had not intended to come back to the lab.

The door creaked open. Otto caught a whiff of magnolia cologne and knew it must be Marianna.

"What's with you, Mare?" David shouted as she approached. "You left our friend uncovered last night. He could have dried out and gone moldy. "

"It wasn't me," said Marianna.

"It better not happen again. I won't let my hard work get trashed by your carelessness."

Stan popped some chocolates into his mouth. Marianna leaned over Otto and peered into his face.

"I had the strangest dream last night," she said, rubbing a bandage on her neck.

"How'd you hurt yourself *there*?" said Stan.

"Could you move so I can work?" said David, nudging Marianna away.

"I'm not sure how it happened. Just a paper cut, I guess. I fell asleep with my head on my desk and my papers all around. There was blood when I woke up."

"Speaking of blood," David said, "what vein do you think this is?"

You'll get used to the bloodlust in time, Otto longed to tell her.

"Could you guys help me here?" said David. "Mare, find this vein in the atlas. I don't know what it is. Do you know what it is?"

"External jugular," said Marianna, without needing to look in the text.

That evening, when he was momentarily alone, Otto raided the lockers outside the anatomy room. Many had been left unlocked. Otto brought several armfuls of lab clothes and dissecting books back to his bed. He stuffed them beneath the sheets, sculpting the bump so that he appeared to still be sleeping. A trick he'd picked up from the grandkids.

When the ruse was complete, Otto glided off to find Marianna. He would have another taste, he thought, and then the two of them could fly away—away from the lab, from Betty and the dreary estate. Perhaps they'd hit Las Vegas. One could amuse oneself there for weeks without having to deal with the sun.

Otto searched Marianna's townhouse, this time wearing a pair of David's scrubs. The place was empty. Otto next scanned the neighborhood and then returned to campus. He fluttered up to the windows of the medical library. Marianna was reading at a carrel in the stacks. Otto threw himself against the glass.

"Come with me," Otto said when Marianna came to the window.

"Listen, Sam. I'm through with you," Marianna said.

Otto swallowed. "Please, just come outside. Just for a moment."

"I have work to do, bud. Leave me alone." Marianna was snarling now, real ugly.

"I think I *will* leave," Otto said. He flapped his wings emphatically as he began to move away. Maybe she'd feel sorry. Maybe she'd allow him one more sip.

"Sam!" called Marianna.

"It's Otto," he said, zipping back to the window.

"You *are* going back to the lab now?"

"I didn't say that."

"You *have* to go back, Sam. We're presenting your neck on Friday." She batted her eyes coquettishly. Otto drooled.

"Will you let me drink again? Will you come away with me when you're through?"

"After Friday," said Marianna. "Just promise you'll stay until Friday."

"I will," Otto said. "Gentleman's honor." He swooped away, flew a loop above the campus, and debated picking up a snack to hold him till the end of the week. But Otto was too courteous to sate himself with an anonymous student. He flew to his estate, hoping to catch his wife in bed with easy prey that he wouldn't feel bad about attacking. Unfortunately, Betty's only companions were the latest Anne Rice novel and a plate of strudel.

In a foul mood, Otto returned to the lab and lay down on the table to wait for Friday.

The next few days were agony for Otto. Despite Marianna's charm, Otto would not have remained until Friday had he not given his word. While Marianna finished the neck, Stan and David peeled the skin off his face. Even worse, they'd begun to talk about taking out his brain.

As soon as the professors see my neck, I'm out of here, Otto vowed. It was Friday afternoon. David and Stan were getting ready for the presentation. Marianna had not yet arrived.

"Where is she?" David was saying, drumming his fingers on the table's metal rim.

"She'll show up," Stan assured.

"What if she fell asleep somewhere? She's seemed overtired lately. Cranky as hell, and have you noticed her eyes?"

"All she needs is Visine and a few days off. We should tell her to go shopping or something. What do girls like to do?"

"You talking about me?"

It was Marianna, charging into the room.

"Oh, boy," David muttered.

"We were just saying how indefatigable you've been lately," Stan said. "I heard you've been pulling all-nighters all week. It's inhuman."

"Indeed," said Marianna. Her eyes shone with the deep red hue of the newly undead.

"Table six, are you ready?" asked Dr. Bloom. She and the other professors approached Otto's bed.

Otto stared at the ceiling and waited for the humiliating show and tell of his body parts to be over. He whiled away the time with thoughts of spangle-clad showgirls, neon lights, and his beloved Marianna, forever within fang's reach.

"Hey—what are you doing?" Marianna glared at Stan and David, who were returning Otto to his plastic and cheesecloth.

"What do you mean? We're done. It's Friday afternoon."

"You're not leaving. I say we start the brain."

"It's the weekend, Mare. I'm tired."

"So, we'll do it fast. Go ask Dr. Bloom for the saw."

Stan and David ran off, muttering under their breath. Marianna removed Otto's wrappings.

"Let's leave now," Otto said. "We'll go to Vegas." Marianna wrinkled her nose. "Or the tropics if you prefer. Someplace with warm nights, hibiscus flowers, and soft pink sand."

"Sorry, Sam, but I have my career to think about," said Marianna. "I worked my whole life to get into medical school. I'm not going to give it up for an old fart like you."

"You're not taking out my brain," said Otto.

"Relax. We'll just peel off the scalp, and then I'll send the boys home—"

"Who are you talking to, Mare?" The guys had returned with the saw. Marianna grabbed it.

"Start scalping," she said. "I've something else to do."

I should have left before. I should leave right now. What am I doing here? thought Otto. Marianna was slicing through his rib cage.

"What are you doing?" David demanded.

"I thought I'd get a head start on the, er, lungs."

"She's crazy," said Stan. "Let's get out of here."

"You're staying!" said Marianna in a tone that gave Stan and his friend no choice. Marianna lowered at Otto. "You're staying," she repeated. Otto sighed. He thought about the days when love had been more important than careers, when women wanted to be swept off their feet. The days when honor, justice, and intellect were valued. Otto did not like this modern world of gimme-gimme grades, money, and sex. In the olden days, your wife would be there after a long night's bloodsucking, greeting you with adoring words and a vigorous back rub before you settled in for a good day's sleep. Betty gave the most luxurious back rubs. Betty Blue, I love you—what was the poem he'd written to propose to her? He'd been such a silly young thing when he proposed, a mere boy of 261.

"Mare, do you really think—?"

Otto snapped back to the present. His front chest wall lay on the floor. The top of his body gaped open like a shoebox without a lid. Marianna's hand was reaching in, grasping the pericardial sac that contained his heart.

"I know what I'm doing," Marianna said. Her right hand held a nasty pair of scissors.

Otto felt his forehead bead with—well, either sweat or formaldehyde. Chopping through skin and muscle was one thing, but mishandling the heart could kill a vampire. A wooden stake through the heart would be murder, Otto knew. He tried to recall what he'd heard about hearts cut out, cut open, and so forth. Otto wished he'd paid more attention to vampire lore. He had always meant to learn more about his cultural background, but then, the stories were always so grizzly.

"This is it, Sam," said Marianna. She jabbed the scissors against the aorta and cut.

"Nooo!" Otto's whole body cried. But there was Marianna holding his heart, and Otto was conscious enough to see it. *We undead really are a hardy bunch*, Otto thought. Marianna poked her finger into what remained of his arm. Otto tried to make his eyes appear even blanker, his body even stiffer than usual.

"I guess that did it," Marianna murmured.

Yesss! She thinks I'm dead now, Otto thought. Marianna would leave, and he could flee to Vegas. Maybe Betty would come too, if she'd still have him. His Betty Blue.

"Can we go now?" said Stan.

"Let's take a look at the heart."

Otto tried to recollect the rules to blackjack while Marianna cleaned the surface of his heart.

"The coronary arteries. Atrium. Atrium. The two ventricles." Marianna displayed the heart to Stan and David, who crowded near. Otto felt proud. His old thumper was pretty amazing.

Marianna slit open the atria. "So beautiful," she said. "Just imagine all that blood, whole liters, and liters of it gushing through these tiny chambers!"

David backed away. "Why don't you go home and get some sleep?"

Marianna glanced toward the window. The sun was beginning to set, and Otto could see that it would be a fabulous night.

"I think I *will* go," Marianna said dreamily. She turned toward Stan. "Here, you take this." She tossed the heart. Stan missed and had to scramble for it under the table.

Dr. Bloom came back. "What's this?" she said. "You've started the heart? I'm impressed that you're working ahead."

Marianna beamed.

"I love the heart," said Dr. Bloom. "That sounds silly, but the heart's so great to see." She took the organ from Stan. "Hardhearted, softhearted, and warmhearted. We're always talking about the heart, but the real thing has no relation to emotions or personality. It's just a pump. Put it in a dish at the right conditions, and it will keep beating. It doesn't need any nervous input, you know. The electrical activity self-generates at the sinoatrial node."

Otto blinked. He couldn't help it. Marianna pursed her lips. Otto's heart gave a thump, or it would have thumped had it still been attached to his body. Marianna had seen his blink. She knew he remained undead.

"Where is the node?" David asked.

I have to get out of here, Otto thought.

"It's not a structure you can see," said Dr. Bloom. "But let me show you where it would be." She took a metal probe from her lab coat pocket.

"Wait. I can show the guys," said Marianna. She took the heart from Dr. Bloom. She was smiling, Otto saw. She was fumbling through a pile of instruments on the table. Otto's heart *really* gave a thump when Marianna selected a slender wooden pointer.

"Don't do it!" Otto cried. He sat up and reached out for the heart with his bony hand. His forehead hit the light that had been poised above his face. His shoulder flopped to the side, so many muscles had been detached. Dr. Bloom, Dan, and Stan were staring, screaming at him, but Marianna stayed calm. She sidled a few feet beyond his grasp and continued speaking.

"The SA node is in the right atrium wall," Marianna was saying. "Right here. Do you see it? In here," she said, eyes gleaming, as she poked the wooden pointer inside.

Melissa Schiffman
Emory University School of Medicine
Class of 1997

A Morning Breath

If I get out of bed now, I can squeeze in that ten-minute morning yoga routine on YouTube. . . . But it feels so nice lying here, sunlight streaming in, sips of coffee warming my body and boosting my heart rate up a notch. If I did anything right in life, it was marrying a man who brings a tumbler of fresh coffee to my bedside every morning. I sip and enjoy the stillness.

The boys must be busy on their devices. Another twenty minutes or so before I have to start rushing them through breakfast, tooth brushing, and out the door to the school bus. My oldest son is almost eleven, closer to the age I started medical school than I am now. (It seems like three hundred years ago that I was working in cadaver lab.) My younger son is in first grade . . . which is having its big Valentine's party tomorrow! Didn't I sign up to send in napkins? When the oldest was in first grade, I did the "doctor mom" thing, coming to his class to teach a lesson about the real heart. I let the kids listen through my stethoscope, and I showed them pictures of the atria, ventricles, and valves in my old anatomy atlas. The kids loved it and, I'll admit, I felt proud to teach them something "cool" and "gross" when the other parents showed up with glitter and glue sticks. Small twinge of guilt that I only volunteered the napkins this year, but this year it's all I feel able to manage. Why are these school events always scheduled at a ridiculous time like 10:45 am on a Tuesday? Don't schools know that parents have to work?

I do what I can.

To do today: maybe yoga. Shower. Get the kids on the school bus. A load of laundry on my way out the door. Then start my real day. Six hours of patients in the primary care clinic. Fifteen minutes for a checkup or urgent problem, thirty minutes for a physical. In the tiny gasps of time in between: refilling scripts, checking labs, and signing medical supply orders and insurance authorization requests. Maybe lunch. Maybe a chance to get to the restroom if I am lucky. Clicking, always clicking away on my EMR, hoping to finish my notes. Maybe typing notes while holding on a phone call (why do patients call with a question about a medicine, but they leave the vial upstairs and have to retrieve it while you wait?), while trying to cram a few bites of lunch, while wondering if I will get out of there in time to get the blasted Valentine's napkins before picking up the kids from their afterschool program.

I take a deep breath.

A "stress management" tip that I read a while back is to take deep breaths along with the patients' inspirations when you auscultate their lungs. The tip is ridiculous and somewhat patronizing. (That is the only time a physician gets to breathe?) Yet, somehow, it helps me to slow down and focus. There is so much to do in a day, but I try to be fully present with each patient. I try to stay mindful that while each visit is just a short blip in my day, it may be an "event" for my patients. They shave their legs or select a pair of socks without holes (or apologize if they have not, as if I care). They prepare lists of questions or consult "Dr. Google" to try to guess what I will say. Maybe they rehearse their stories ahead of time, how they will gently lead into the reason for the appointment. "Doc, I know you'll be mad at me. I never got the colonoscopy we talked about last year, and now the blood is in my stool again." Or "It's so silly, probably just stress, but I'm having sweats at night, and sometimes I get dizzy." They sit before me on the cold table, their expressions so often betraying shame or fear, dismay at their body's failings, longing for reassurance or a cure. I understand the weight of this strange job that deals in sickness and health, life, and death. Mostly in fifteen-minute intervals.

I remember a mentor in med school trying to dissuade me from a career in primary care. "Won't you get bored of treating colds all day?" she said. The truth is, after twenty years, I am not bored. Primary care is so much more than "colds." And even a cold is not a cold. It could be a patient who secretly fears that she has lung cancer, or an elderly man with an exacerbation of heart failure, or a new mother who, now that you mention it, has been having crying jags every afternoon while the baby naps and could use someone to talk to.

I love the variety and the intimacy of the problems that are placed before me. I feel privileged to peer so deeply into the essence of humanity . . . the lumps and boils and sore throats, the fears and anxieties; all the mental and physical imperfections that make us human. Maybe we doctors enter this profession, in large part, to try to defend ourselves and our loved ones against illness and pain. The longer we practice, the more we understand that many ailments cannot be prevented or cured. We become more comfortable with limitations and uncertainties. Hopefully, we sharpen our ability to at least soothe, or to serve as a witness. So often, a patient will thank me just for listening. I hope that whatever I do, it helps.

I just wish I had more help with the rest of it, not the doctoring, but the unrelenting scut parts of the job that threaten to drain me dry. So much paperwork. Red tape and logistics. ICD and CPT codes. The work absence letters and FMLA forms. Not to mention finishing up the day's office notes late at night in the back room of my house, when I should be reading a novel, or joining my husband for a glass of wine, or preparing Valentine's snacks for the next day. (Will the boys notice if I don't? Will their friends' moms have artsy little muffins ready for them at tomorrow's breakfast? If I hug them extra-tight, will my sons of a doctor know that a healthy, beating heart means so much more than a sugary emoji?)

I do what I can . . . for my patients, my family . . . and if there is a tiny bit left, for myself.

The bedroom door creaks open. "Mommy, will you make me oatmeal?"

Simultaneously, a text from the on-call service. "Patient's fingerstick is 426 this morning, wants to know how much insulin to take." I look at the clock. I guess YouTube yoga is not going to happen. I put down my coffee and lie back in bed, for one last moment. I take a deep breath in, expanding my lungs, filling my belly, and stretching my toes. I guess this counts as savasana, the yoga position known as corpse pose. It will have to do. I arise again to start my day.

Melissa Schiffman, M.D.
Pediatrics

POSTLUDE

Perhaps we crossed paths on a street corner . . .
What do I know about you?
Only that you set your affairs in order
So that my life would one day cross your death
Signaling the start of my new career
I fear that you will cry out
When I cut your hand or your breast
But when you don't and there is only stillness
I probe some more.
I'm angry at your body
Too many arteries, muscles, and veins
Can I tease sensations from these nerves?
Where are your memories if not in this brain?
Slowly it dawns on me
That death was a moment of passage
A skull without a brain can't continue to be you
And however hard I work, I'll never dissect your soul.
In this room full of cadavers
Lives lived well or not, the struggles are over
Not life nor death here, but profound quiet Do I feel as I hover
and uncover layer by layer this body
learning
listening
and
feeling
That this, above all is a room full of gifts.

Lisa M. Gibbs
Stanford University School of Medicine
Class of 1996

MEMOIR (2020)

By now we have crossed paths many times . . .
What do I know about you?
Only what you remember and choose to tell
So that I can provide comfort and hope
Signaling the rest of our time together

I fear that you will retreat
When I dispense of niceties and focus on what matters
And when you are still, either vacant or stalwart
I probe some more.

What dares lead us to darkness?
Lost moments, or glimmers and shimmers
They are there, then they are not
Where are your memories if not in this brain?

Slowly it dawns on me
That life is a moment of passage
You, at this moment, are a collage of all moments before
And no matter what Time takes; it'll never take your soul

We grieve what we cannot cure
lives lived well or not
the struggles are slowly fading . . .
In this transit between the life we know
and life we do not know
I find profound quiet

As I hover and uncover
layer by layer
this Person

learning
listening
and
˙feeling

That this journey, above all, is a room full of gifts.

Lisa M. Gibbs, M.D.
Geriatrics & Family Medicine

SOMETHING FOR JOHN

He walked in the room
surrounded by adult, protecting arms . . . three pairs to be exact.

We were faces wearing lab coats, poised at notebooks.

We didn't know what to expect when his tiny body could be seen through their legs.

But we must have frightened him because he buried his hairless head in Grandma's knee. I ventured, "Hi, John," and smiled.

Tony gave him three pieces of candy, but he never spoke a word—or left Grandma's lap.

His mom told us about the cancer and how sick her baby was,

And she told us how alone the two healthy ones felt. And we could see how strong she was, and scared.

A four-year-old doesn't know he's dying—he just doesn't like "ouchies!"

But Mom knows—so does Grandma.

So did we.

After they left, I cried—a few of us did.

Yes, we can support each other, but still, we feel inadequate.

Someday that doctor may be me—diagnosing and treating the very diseases I'm furiously trying to keep straight in my head now.

I'm scared.

The fears of uncertainty, inadequacy, and failure riddle me.

I don't feel secure relying on "process of elimination" diagnoses or "trial and error" therapy, but sometimes . . . it's the best you have. Somehow, any resentment or envy of missed opportunities nonmedical students enjoy diminished today.

Perhaps I'll only live 80 percent of the dreams I dream, but there promises an infinity of encounters I may taste that others will never experience —like the tears of today.

And there may be another little boy who can live my other 20 percent. . . .

Another John . . . who can enjoy something more than just candy and smiles.

Shelby Lynette Clay
Northeastern Ohio Universities College of Medicine
Class of 1997

FOCUSING

When our medical school class encountered "John" for the first time, it made a huge impact on many of us.

So many times during medical school and residency, I would become frustrated or discouraged because of the countless hours of studying, the thousands of nuggets of information I tried to store in my brain, and the sacrifices of time and a social life in my prime years. Sometimes, I even resented my choice to pursue medicine. Sometimes, even now, I question why I do what I do. Unappreciative patients, demanding families, grouchy consultants, and unreasonable administration seem to be everywhere. It's hard to focus on the blessings when focusing on the disapproval.

Instead, I choose to focus on the blessings:

ENCOUNTERS
But then I remembered "John" or so many of the other individual faces and stories I have encountered over the years. They have shaped me, molded me, and created the physician I am today.

I remember the person I diagnosed with leukemia because of his occupation. I recall the old man with nine fingers and a positive TB test who grinned when I snuck him chocolate ice cream after rounds and made the front page of the paper the morning after he was discharged because he blew up his apartment complex while smoking on the oxygen I had prescribed for him. I remember the positive attitude of the young person who I learned the art of lumbar punctures on due to his intrathecal chemotherapy

34

three times a week . . . and when he came into the emergency department to teach me about tumor lysis syndrome—the hard way. I remember the first time I saw a Chovstek's sign from hypercalcemia in an eight-year-old . . . and the second time years later because of malnutrition—both in a first-world country.

PRIVILEGES

Being a doctor of medicine is a privilege. I do not want to lose sight of that or take it for granted. I am the one blessed by blessing others.

I acknowledge the fact that people tell me things in confidence that nobody else knows, speak to me kindly when I know if we met in a dark alley it would be a different conversation, and let me intimately examine them when they just met me and don't know me at all.

I am present when a little life is discovered through the mama's urine when she comes in for a "stomach bug."

I am sitting on the stool at the side of the bed explaining the life-threatening situation a patient is facing and the options we need to work through right now with their family crying on the other end of the cell phone.

I hold the stethoscope to the chest of someone's grandmother and hear nothing as I stare at the straight line on the monitor and glance at my watch for the time of death.

I offer a small box of crunchy tissues to the weeping parents of a teenager who didn't live to make it to the trauma bay after the bullet struck his chest outside of the fast-food restaurant downtown at two in the morning.

HUMILITY

I hold myself to a higher standard, to set an example, and to be who I am called to be. But I need to remember that I am still just a person doing a job, my job, to the best of my ability. I fashion my motto after that of Theodore Roosevelt when he said, "Do what you can, with what you have, where you are."

I try to be strong, decisive, clear, and hopeful when I explain the reasons behind my tests and recommendations. I believe that compliance depends on comprehension and trust.

I share a smile, let a kid listen to his own heartbeat with my stethoscope, joke a little with my patients, give a hug to a family member, or pray with a family when it's appropriate.

I strive to see the good in people and give the benefit of the doubt, even when most others are cynical.

I hope to make a difference in the lives of my patients. Their families. My colleagues. My hospital staff. My hospital family.

I hold myself accountable to anyone who sees my actions, hears my voice, or knows my heart.

I am not better than others because of my education, my degree, or my profession.

I am a person—hard working, conscientious, dedicated, concerned, and compassionate—but just a person.

I tell my staff in the emergency department to call my Shelby . . . or Doctor Shelby if they prefer.

After all, I was Shelby long before I was Doctor.

ACCEPTANCE

Life and death, health and illness, celebrations and grieving, hope and despair, and successes and failures. This is the dichotomy of medicine and, in fact, the dichotomy of our existence. One doesn't occur without the other. We must learn to thrive in the midst of them all.

During this time of uncertainty and unknown with the COVID-19 pandemic, we are face to face with all the above simultaneously each and every day. Following the earthquake in Haiti in January 2010, while tending to patients in a quaint Haitian hospital, the dichotomy was ever present. Even with the most mundane hospital shift, the potential for each extreme exists. We do not get to choose which side of the line we are assigned to at any given time.

We must function with humility *during* any season when we are privileged *with* patient encounters *and* we must continue to thrive through the acceptance *of* the outcomes in order to see and experience the blessings.

Shelby Clay-Rogers, M.D.
Emergency Medicine

THE WINDING ROAD AHEAD

I've given a lot of thought about what it means to become a doctor. Words cannot do justice to all the complexities of medical school, but I'll do my best to relay to you some of the highlights of my experiences thus far. The journey through medical school is thought provoking, to say the least. The road through the first two years has had many curves.

I believe that I will forever recall the first day of gross anatomy. Like one's graduation from high school or college or any other milestone in one's life, it is an indelible memory—with me for a lifetime. It is a rite of passage, an "initiation" per se, into medicine. It was striking to look around at the sea of white lab coats. We were the future. We were going to be doctors. My God—it was finally *real*. Over the course of a semester, we had begun the transformation from timid students to future clinicians. I remember our apprehension that first day when our lab group removed the covering from the cadaver. It was all new and frightening. Throughout the year, some students and I engaged in discussions regarding our varying philosophies about death. It was somewhat surprising to all of us that we could separate ourselves from our surroundings in the anatomy lab. Not with irreverence, but with some degree of familiarity, by the semester's close in December, we were able to dissect with the faint chimes of classical music or Christmas carols in the background.

Through countless hours of biochemistry, histology, physiology, neuroanatomy, and so on, I discovered that medical school was more than just books or labs. As I became involved with the school's community activities, I realized that I was becoming an activist. The realization set in that I could one day be a role model in the community. It was an empowering time in my life. I volunteered at a local homeless shelter, did an internship at an AIDS clinic in North Philadelphia, and participated in a program for inner-city elementary students designed to build self-esteem. My naivete was stripped away somewhat on my third visit to the elementary school. I noticed that one of my students was withdrawn that day. Thinking back to my own childhood, I attributed his behavior to, perhaps, an argument with a parent or a sibling the evening before. After some time, "Jeremy" looked at me and quietly said, "My friend died yesterday."

"Died?" I asked.

"How did your friend die?"

"He was shot," was the reply.

I could say nothing; I felt powerless. I had so much to learn about this world, a new violent world that I had not known at seven years of age. I asked myself where I fit in as a future doctor. Could I make a difference in the community?

My feelings of helplessness eroded a bit sometime later when, at the homeless shelter, I met a young man who had come to see a clinic doctor about a headache. Knowing little about the physical exam, I was instructed to record the patient's history. "Orlando" had a thirteen-year history of cocaine addiction. I asked him if he would like to be enrolled in a rehabilitation program. To my surprise—a sigh of relief followed by a resounding "yes, please." With childlike enthusiasm, I worked with the staff to set up an appointment for him. He thanked me, and I had a sense of accomplishment. The doctor at the clinic told me that I was naive, that the chance the young man would "come clean" was very slim. "Most people enter rehab and fail twelve times," he said. "You're idealistic." Unbroken, I told him that I hoped to retain my idealism throughout my career. I had faith. When I last checked, "Orlando" was still drugfree.

In the second year, I became self-absorbed. My attention shifted from the community to myself. I, along with several classmates, developed an incurable case of MSS—"Medical Student Syndrome." My occasional cough was undoubtedly bronchogenic carcinoma, and my lower back pain was certainly a dissecting aortic aneurysm. I realized that the hypochondriac in me had taken full hold when, during a cystic fibrosis (CF) lecture, I became convinced that I had an undiagnosed case of CF. I found myself licking my skin to see if I tasted salty. When I glanced to my right, I noticed that a fellow student was doing the same! Enough. I had to conquer this.

You begin to think that everyone is ill. The prognosis seems so dismal, and you simply cannot bear to read another heart-wrenching case history that invariably concludes, " . . . and the patient expired." It is difficult not to become engrossed in illness and death. Slowly, though, we've all begun to deal with MSS. It is only time and experience that will quell this syndrome.

It is the trend this year to define your clinical aptitude by your performance in the clinical workshops. A good friend of mine disclosed to me that she had fainted during the IV workshop. "How can I be a doctor?" she asked. I assured her that she was not the first med student to feel queasy upon inserting an IV, and I reassured her that this was no reflection on her ability to become a good clinician. Of course, I know that the same thing could happen to me, and I often ponder what my own obstacles will be.

Eagerly looking forward to my own future, I have reduced my expectations of what doctors can do. My initial Godlike impression has wavered somewhat. I've learned that much of medicine is an educated guess, and sometimes doctors, like everyone else, must say, "I don't know." As I move closer to obtaining the coveted MD degree, I still have a great respect and admiration for the work that physicians do; however, I no longer place them on a pedestal because as I move forward to join the ranks, I am apprehensive about standing on one. Becoming a doctor is a privilege, and I hope to carry with me some of the naivete and enthusiasm with which I entered medical school. I am excited that I will never stop learning, that the patient will become my teacher, and that the road will continue to wind in endless turns.

Lisa Christopher
Hahnemann University School of Medicine
Class of 1997

Vulnerability and a Twenty-Five-Year Journey of the Unknown

"I don't feel it." Silence and then an audible gasp among them. Five students peered at my physical examination skills as I tried to locate the dorsalis pedis pulse in one of the students on which I was demonstrating the vascular examination. "Is that possible?" one of them said out loud. "Do some people not have the pulse, or is it possible that you just sometimes cannot find it?" They wanted to know.

That was a moment, a teachable one that I stopped to reflect upon: the concept of "not knowing." I realized that these young students assumed that senior faculty must always know the answer, feel the pulse, hear the murmur, and find the infection. I realized that it was so important to explain why saying "I don't know" is not only truthful, but also imperative for the best healthcare.

I eventually located the pulse, lateral to where it would be expected to be located, allowing me to talk about physiologic and anatomic variations. It also allowed me to remind students that stating that we see or feel something that we don't can have negative consequences. Imagine, for example, noting that there was no murmur when in fact there was. This misses the opportunity for further exploration to find the root cause of such a finding.

Perhaps it is twenty-three years as a licensed physician that allows me the latitude to have the confidence to be vulnerable. Vulnerability is something we don't teach enough in healthcare, but that should be required more often.

40

Since I was a medical student beginning my journey to becoming a physician, we began to have conversations about the principles and practices of medicine. Still in its infancy, this concept was unusual, and even in the late 1990s, the top-down approach to healthcare was evident. Senior physicians have all the answers. Junior physicians need to learn those answers. And the medical students are at the bottom of that food chain.

It comes as an irony to me that some of the most stellar physicians that I have seen and now model myself after are those who have had the confidence to say, "I don't know." It's the starting point for a conversation, for acquiring new knowledge, and for realizing what is and is not known about certain conditions.

I chose to pursue rheumatology subspecialty training, and that is likely not an accidental choice. I have always loved immunology, and I had the privilege of seeing the science of immunology meld into clinical practice when in the late 1990s, medications were developed to target specific portions of the immune response. I literally saw people walk out of their wheelchairs. It was a time where we celebrated and realized that we could bring into bedside practice the knowledge gained at the lab bench. I chose to pursue an academic career, but rheumatology is a humbling subspecialty. For all the strides over the past three decades, there is so very much we still don't know. In my particular subspecialty, autoimmune inflammatory muscle disease, more broadly known as "myositis," we still do not have any pharmaceutical treatments that are specifically indicated to treat myositis aside from prednisone, and we borrow all of them without precision. Saying, "We don't know," is the first step to realizing what we need to know, and it heralds a future of precision medicine, which then further leads to personalized medicine.

What a metamorphosis these last twenty-five years have been since I wrote my original essay. On a personal level, the changes have been immense. I am now a mother to two growing boys, and I have been married for nearly twenty-two years to my then-boyfriend of two years when I wrote my first essay in *Becoming Doctors*. I assumed that by the time I had doubled my age, I would have double the wisdom. Perhaps on some level that is true, but in other ways, I feel like the more I learn, the more I realize what I still do not know. And perhaps it is this phase of my career that allows me to feel comfort in the not knowing. I write this as we all battle a pandemic, and we realize for everything we learn about the coronavirus enveloping the planet, there is yet something else that we do not understand. It is a virus of paradoxes. It is our teacher, not only uncovering healthcare disparities, but also immunologic features of infections, the chance to demonstrate how worldwide collaborations work well, and it assisted us in the shepherding of the era of telemedicine.

The tone of the world today is one of uncertainty and unrest. The glimpse into the inequities in marginalized communities and lack of access to healthcare and basic human necessities that I had as a young medical student have been magnified. Through the lens of demands for social justice, I see clearly that I must be part of the solution to help erode a tiered system of healthcare in the United Sates.

So, I take a deep breath and look forward to the next twenty-five years, at which point I hope to have looked back on the successes of the healthcare system, the birth of personalized healthcare and big data, and my own fulfilling career, but also to the excitement of realizing that trainees just beginning will have yet another new world to journey of things yet unknown.

Lisa Christopher Stine, M.D.
Rheumatology

THE ROLE OF
UNCERTAINTY AS A TOOL
OF DISCOVERY IN MY LIFE

"Negative Capability—That is when man is capable of being in uncertainties, mysteries, doubts, without any irritable reaching after fact and reason . . ." English poet and physician John Keats wrote these words 203 years ago to describe what he thought was the "quality [which] went to form a Man of Achievement." I was excited to learn that our topic in human context this week was "Uncertainty in Medicine." Through my undergraduate studies in philosophy and literature, I came to discover that I could attain a heightened state of awareness when I could allow myself to remain in a state of uncertainty and perplexity over an issue. The aspect of uncertainty that I find to be the most intriguing is its potential use as a unique kind of tool for discovery.

I have found that often when a situation or issue causes some kind of unpleasant feeling within me, such as regret, worry, or fear, this is a cue for me to stop and ask the following two questions: "What is this situation about, really?" and "What am I supposed to learn from this?" I don't ask these two questions of anyone or anything in particular. I guess if I were forced to pinpoint exactly of what or of whom I was asking these two questions, I would say that I am partly asking God, partly my subconscious, and partly my feelings themselves. I ask these questions quietly, aloud a few times, and then I just wait. I wait with a sense of uncertainty and perplexity. I wait to see what thoughts and realizations begin to pop up in my head over the next few hours or days in regard to that issue. Amazingly, thoughts and realizations begin to surface inside of me within a few hours or days after I have posed these questions. These realizations usually help me to see something new about the original issue or situation, and it's usually some aspect I had not even considered before.

One of the best words I have found to describe this experience is *serendipity:* "An aptitude for making desirable discoveries by accident," as defined in *Webster's.* I try to keep from actively pursuing an answer since I have found out that course of thought usually causes me to focus upon conclusions reached using the parameters of my biases, limited knowledge, and immediate feelings about the issue at hand. In these instances, the unpleasant feelings of regret, worry, or anxiety usually persist, almost as if they were attempting to persuade me to look deeper and longer at my situation.

The following is an example of how I was able to attain and use a state of uncertainty to resolve a conflict recently.

When I heard that my medical school had a rugby team, I grew excited over the idea of joining. A few days before the first practice, however, I realized what a great deal of study material was piling up for me each day, and I felt anxiety over the thought of losing valuable study time by going out for rugby. A decision to not go out for the team was easy at first. "I'll simply go jogging and lift weights in my free time to stay in shape and get a diversion from studying, "I thought. Yet a short while later, I found myself feeling regret and anxiety over not taking the opportunity to participate in a school sport like rugby. I thought to myself, "This is probably the last time before I graduate that I'll have a chance to play on a rugby team." After flipflopping back and forth many times between these two opposing conclusions, I found that I was still unable to make a decision I felt good about. After several days of growing frustration, I suddenly remembered to put into practice my "two questions." "What is this about, really?" and "What am I supposed to learn from this?" I asked myself. I then let myself remain in a patient state of wonder and observance.

A short while later, I had a sudden realization about what the real issue behind my frustration was. I had never been able to become the great football player that I had worked so fervently to become throughout two years of high school and two years of college ball. My desire to play rugby was to a large extent an extension of these curtailed efforts of my youth. Yet, I recalled, years ago I had promised myself that if I didn't make it as a star athlete in life, I would set out to discover what field my talent actually lay in and that, if I found it, I would pursue it with the same intensity as football.

I realized that I was now in training to become a member of a select group of people who hold the title of MD and that my being here showed I possessed some degree of talent in the area of academics, as well as a unique opportunity for achievement. Of course! I needed to direct my thwarted drive to make it as a professional athlete into making it as a professional physician and healer!

Dr. Smith (not his real name), one of our group discussion panelists on Wednesday, described an experience of his that seemed to parallel mine, in that he too was able to use a time of uncertainty to step back and discover a larger perspective to his circumstances. One of his patients called him one evening to complain of a pain that was preventing him from getting to sleep. It sounded to Dr. Smith as if the symptoms were probably not serious and he told his patient not to worry about it that evening. The patient died at home shortly afterward. Dr. Smith spent a week in depression and severe anguish over his decision. He told our class that he flipflopped back and forth, going from, on one hand, the conclusion that he was an incompetent doctor and should leave the field of medicine, to the other conclusion that he made the best decision he could have under the circumstances and he should not feel guilty about it. Neither of these competing ideas, however, helped to quell his anguish. Finally, after a week, he said, a sudden realization "came to him." "I suddenly realized," he told us, "hey, I am *human*. When did I forget that and begin to think I was incapable of error?" Dr. Smith was able to come to see a larger underlying issue to his situation, which encompassed and transcended his two earlier antagonistic conclusions. His realization helped him to transcend his anxiety and to begin to approach his practice of medicine with a truer sense of his own potential for error and with more realistic expectations of his own capabilities.

At this point, I am uncertain whether I have adequately written about the role "uncertainty" can or should play in medicine and life. Yet I am keeping an open mind to the possibility that I may soon receive further realizations, which may help me transcend the conclusions I have already come to about this subject.

James Eric Bermudez
Uniformed Services University of the Health Sciences
F. Edward Hebert School of Medicine
Class of 1998

The Physician's Optimal Role in the Healing Process

One of my favorite quotes as pertains to the practice of medicine is the following:

> Understand that you are a channel through which healing moves, and that you are contacting the healing force within your patients . . . You will have awakened the physician within them . . . and sent them on their way to cure themselves.
> —Gladys McGarey, MD, from *The Physician Within You*

An important realization that most of us physicians come to at some point in our practice of medicine is that the healing process is not the result of the medications we prescribe or the surgical procedures that we accomplish. At best, when used properly and judiciously, medicines and surgical interventions are adjuncts that can serve to facilitate the healing process for our patients . . . a process that results from the inherent healing systems and capacities that lie within the patients themselves.

The physician who desires to best serve his or her patients must acknowledge, respect, and seek to align with—and work with—these innate processes.

When we are truthful with ourselves, as physicians, we come to realize that the role that we play in the healing process is a peripheral one and not a central one.

Nurses, medical technicians, and doctors alike all receive regular reminders during our trainings and our careers regarding the importance of the "five Rs": the right patient, the right drug, the right dose, the right timing, and the right route (of administration).

If any of these guiding factors is neglected or violated (e.g., wrong patient, wrong drug, wrong dose, wrong timing, or wrong route), the outcome can be harmful and destructive.

The drugs and surgical instruments that we wield can certainly pose dangers when used in a non-judicious and improper manner, and they can detrimentally interfere with the human body's innate health and healing capacities. This fact underscores the simple reality that the cause of healing does not originate within a pill or a scalpel blade—although, again, these can be helpful tools to enhance and promote healing if used carefully and wisely . . . and only when absolutely necessary.

"First, do no harm" is the prime directive of medicine. It is a precept that is neglected by us physicians at our own peril—and at the peril of the health of our patients, as well. This "first rule" of medicine is a guiding principle that instructs us to be minimalists with regard to interventions (medications, surgeries, and other procedures), and it reminds us to be ever vigilant against our human capacity to, at times, clumsily meddle or interfere with natural processes in excessive, unnecessary, or even harmful ways.

***

When a patient comes to us with an illness or other malady, we must realize and continually remember that our role involves seeking to facilitate whatever innate healing capacities that currently exist and that are currently at work within the patient himself or herself and in the least invasive and least potentially harmful manner as possible.

Nearly every category of medication has a spectrum of options, which range from least potentially toxic to most potentially toxic.

For example, in the category of pain-relieving medications, aspirin and acetaminophen (TYLENOL) may be considered to be on the lower end of the "potentially toxic" scale, while morphine and fentanyl are certainly on the higher end of that spectrum.

Of course, since human physiology varies from patient to patient, even acetaminophen or aspirin could be seriously harmful for certain individuals, such as those with underlying liver dysfunction or an aspirin allergy.

Careful history-taking and physical examination skills, as well as competence in our diagnosis, treatment, and referral-making skills, prove invaluable for physicians as we seek to avoid the many potential treatment pitfalls that exist and help our patients achieve the successful health outcomes that both they and we desire.

Acknowledging the individual differences and unique characteristics of each of our patients informs our ability to help to potentially put them in closer touch with their own inner healer, their innate healing capacities.

***

Knowing when to avoid and abstain from prescribing medications or procedures is just as crucial and important as our ability to properly discern when to recommend, and how to properly utilize, these interventions.

Rest and observation are two all-important facilitators of healing, and every doctor knows that during our patient encounters, we must carefully determine, and weigh in our minds, when these approaches are medically indicated and when they should be the sole recommendations that we give to our patients.

Furthermore, the physician who seeks after excellence in his or her practice works to become competent and skilled at instructing his or her patients regarding selfcare, home remedies, and natural healing methods when these simple (and very often nontoxic) approaches are appropriate and indicated, as well.

***

As aspiring physicians, in our undergraduate studies and during medical school, we become familiar with the concept of homeostasis—an important physiological phenomenon observed in living organisms throughout the plant and animal kingdoms.

A manifestation of this phenomenon in human beings is the natural, innate capacities of restoration, rejuvenation, and healing that are at work in our bodies on a continual basis.

When we become ill or injured, those healing forces go into overdrive to repair the damage, to oust the foreign invaders (bacteria, viruses, parasites, etc.), or to otherwise relieve the malady in other needed ways.

A cast and/or perhaps a surgery, as examples, which are utilized to stabilize or set a broken bone . . . or antibiotics that are given to reduce the high bacterial load involved in an infection . . . or anti-inflammatory medications that are given to reduce excessive inflammatory responses . . . can all be used to help to enable, guide, and augment the healing process.

But, again, it bears repeating that the healing that occurs is the result of the innate processes and systems that exist within the patients themselves.

Neither the drugs, nor the interventions, nor the mere presence of us mighty doctors ourselves have actually "caused" the act of healing that takes place in our patients.

Believe it or not, we physicians are prone to forgetting this fact more often than you might think . . . and more often than many of us would like to admit!

Yet, respect for the natural processes of the human body is one of the hallmarks of the mature and self-reflective physician, and it also happens to be the true meaning of practicing "patient-centered" care and "patient-centered" medicine.

What's more, this sense of respect for the human body's important natural capacities also happens to be a fundamental component of competence, as well as long-term career success and sustainability for us physicians in this field we call the "practice" of medicine.

I am grateful to my teachers and mentors who have taught me this important truth along my path over the years.

In addition, I am also appreciative for every one of my patients who, perhaps unknowingly, serve to repeatedly remind me of this simple but eternally elusive principle during my interactions and encounters with them.

James Eric Bermudez, M.D.
Family Medicine & Aerospace Medicine

GROSS ANATOMY

I never saw the movie
but those two words alone made me
shiver as an entering medical student
I envisioned myself: hand shaking, stomach turning
Nightmares of walking mummies
But when I finally faced you
I was surprised to discover beauty
It was like a present waiting to be unwrapped
Revealing all your glory
Like treasures deep under the ocean
Only sometimes I could not find them. I was not looking in the right place.
I was not careful enough . . . but on the rare occasion that I did, I felt proud
and grateful
Thank you
for teaching me where the vagus nerve lies
for teaching me patience

Thank you for showing me a part of what it means to be human

Lisa L. Wong
University of Hawaii John A. Burns School of Medicine
Class of 1996

TRADING PLACES

"Excuse me," I said. I hated interrupting my patient as she was giving her history, but I abruptly stood up and closed the door behind me so I could get to the trash can around the corner and throw up. I discovered I was pregnant just a few weeks before, the very morning my father passed away. It was too late to tell him the good news—his first grandchild was on the way. He was an endocrinologist, trained at the Mayo Clinic and much loved by his large panel of patients. I had joined his busy private practice six months earlier, and he was thrilled to have me on board. I, on the other hand, was distracted with my search for a house after completing my residency and fellowship in Washington, D.C., and moving back home. I would see a few patients of his and then flit off to meet our realtor. When he was diagnosed with gastric cancer six months later, I had no choice but to "drink from the fire hose" since he could no longer work. He had well over two thousand patients, and every one of them was new to me. As I took their heavy chart in my hands to greet each one, they would offer their condolences. Some of them had been with him since he started out in 1979. It was obvious how much they missed him, but I had no time to grieve as I tried to decipher his distinctive slanted handwriting. What were this patient's problem list, past medications, and laboratory results? I attempted to fit the puzzle pieces together while listening to their concerns and learning about the rhythms of their family and work life.

Stepping into my father's large shoes was no easy feat. First of all, I looked too young. Would these patients trust me? Perhaps I should cut my hair short or wear pantyhose. Even after my training, I felt unprepared to manage a business. I made the decision to discontinue the chemistry labs in his office. A decade later, I navigated through a myriad of electronic medical record choices. One of the most difficult decisions was to switch to a concierge practice and bid many patients farewell. Would he have approved?

Gradually, I came to realize how fortunate I was to inherit this thriving practice. His office was designed by my uncle, who was asked to structure the large, welcoming exam rooms similar to the Mayo. The black and white photos my father developed in his own makeshift darkroom still hang on the walls. Workflow was efficient and friendly. Patients became my ohana as we shared struggles and victories together through health challenges and chronic diseases. I found myself learning my father's diagnostic and treatment style as well as how he administered gentle guidance through each of these patients. My diabetic patients would inform me, "Your father used to tell me to eat cucumbers and tomato instead of mango and pineapple."

It would be many years before I could let go of the trinkets and reminders of Dad in his office. It was many years before I moved into his office space. I finally made the transition after my medical assistant's persistent urging, but it took a while before I started to feel comfortable in his leather chair.

Since he's been gone, pharmaceutical representatives no longer offer free pens. Health insurance companies require justification with pre-authorizations for medications. We no longer write on a prescription pad since we can e-prescribe to the pharmacy. Physicians don't see their patients who are admitted to the hospital since they have hospitalists for that. What would he have thought of telemedicine in the time of COVID-19?

Although the landscape has changed, there are some things that have remained constant over the past twenty years. Our two medical assistants who are like gold. Familiarity of our patients' preferences and rhythms. The quest for scientific knowledge and best practices. My role as advocate and cheerleader. Laughter that punctuates our days. What would Dad have thought?

My mother reassures me that he would be proud.

Lisa L. Wong, M.D.
Endocrinology

NOT JUST ANOTHER NIGHT ON CALL

At major university medical centers, there are many layers of physician responsibility for a patient's care; first is the attending physician and then often a fellow (a doctor in more advanced training). There is usually at least one resident on the team, sometimes two. Finally, there is the medical student. At my medical school, we have no fellows and only a small contingent of residents. Most of the time, it is just the attending physician and the student. Sometimes, this places a large burden of responsibility on the student, but I believe this is an advantage to our program. It is in situations like the one I faced when I met John Karlson (not his real name) that I have grown the most as a physician-in-training.

I have often wondered about death, about what makes the last breath that a person draws any different from the millions they have drawn previously. As a medical student who has spent thousands of hours poring over textbooks and listening to lectures, it is easy to get caught up in the science of death. "What would that myocardial tissue look like under a microscope?" I've pondered. That's why it was easy to dissociate myself the night my attending physician phoned to tell me that he was admitting a patient with end-stage cancer. "Well, this could be an interesting case," I thought, "a chance to test some of my skills."

When I met John in the emergency room, he was with his wife and son. He was an elderly male and clearly in a lot of pain. His wife and son were distraught. It had become too difficult for them to manage his care at home. My attending physician had told me that comfort care would be the treatment goal for this dying patient, but I could see that the family had not yet come to grips with John's condition. I now had two goals: control Mr. Karlson's pain and help the family understand what was happening.

As I stood in the cubicle with John and his family, I felt alone. My attending physician was just a phone call away, and I was in an emergency room surrounded by excellent physicians and nursing staff. If John were to start having seizures or stop breathing, help was at hand. However, in regard to helping the family, the responsibility was mine, and I was definitely alone.

I spoke with my attending physician and decided on a protocol for treating Mr. Karlson. Then I was up for the rest of the night making certain that his needs for comfort were met, but mostly talking things over with Mr. Karlson's wife and son.

John hung on for a week. During that time, I would check on him many times a day. His wife or his son—often both—were always there. I answered questions, and we would talk. Sometimes, we would just sit, and I became quite close to them. When there was a problem or a question that arose, the Karlsons would ask to speak with me. In their eyes, I was the caregiver, though they knew well that I was only a student. They kept telling me how much I helped, how much comfort I gave them. Somehow, though, I felt totally worthless. I wished for a magic wand that I could wave, but medicine doesn't have one. I know now that wasn't what the Karlsons wanted; they wanted a shoulder to lean on, someone to listen and answer a few questions, and that I could do. Mrs. Karlson told me repeatedly that she would remember me forever. I hope so. I will carry her and her husband in my heart for all the years that I practice medicine, and I will be forever thankful for what they taught me about compassion. This is the kind of lesson I'm not sure you could get in a setting other than the one we have here in my program.

The night came when John's breathing changed. He was gasping and would stop breathing for what seemed an eternity. I didn't think about the changes in the color of his skin or those occurring in his brain. His wife held one hand, and I held the other, and I watched this woman who had loved her husband nearly twice as long as I had been alive. I thought about the loneliness of losing someone you've loved for so long.

Inexplicably, his body decided that the breath he now took was to be his last. Mrs. Karlson kissed him on the forehead and began to cry. "What am I going to do now?" she sobbed. I wept quietly with her, but I didn't know the answer. I stood with Mrs. Karlson for a while—maybe half an hour, I don't really remember. Then I called my wife to tell her that I loved her and that I wanted to grow old with her.

Joshua Weil
University of Illinois College of Medicine at Rockford
Class of 1995

LIFE TURNS ON A DIME

The indelible memory of the early hours of October 9, 2017, remains—and will always be—the sound of my then fifteen-year-old daughter, Sophie, screaming at the other end of my wife's cell phone. Breathless and out of control, I knew the fire was upon them, and it was possible I was listening to my daughter dying two miles away from me. I was completely helpless to do anything. I'm an emergency physician with nearly twenty-five years of experience. I'm trained to handle life and death scenarios, to be decisive, and to avoid panic, but all I could do was tell Sophie to slow down her breathing, that I was with her, and that she was going to be okay. I did not actually know if that was true.

I will always remember October 8 as an odd day. It was incredibly hot. I had tried to get some work done on the little barn for our goats, but it was too intolerable, so I gave up. I found myself in our "casita," the little outbuilding where my wife had consigned most of my sports memorabilia, old yearbooks, and photos from my past. I pulled out my time trial road bike I'd ridden thousands of miles training and competing in endurance triathlons. I cleaned it, lubed it, and then set it up on the rollers, promising myself that I would get back into riding and start training again. I found myself flipping through some of those old yearbooks, reminiscing about friends and my past. I'm a very sentimental person and I'm rooted in my history, which holds meaning and has always brought me comfort and a degree of peace. While I spent an hour or so looking through photos and letters, I never could have imagined that it would be the last time I would see any of those treasures from my past.

I was scheduled for the overnight shift that Sunday, and as had been my habit, I tried to go down for a nap around 6:00 PM. It was hot and windy, and our power would go off periodically, shutting down the fan in our

56

room and the air conditioner, making it very hard to sleep. A little after 9:00 PM, I gave up, wandered out of our bedroom, and resigned myself to a shift where I might be a little sleep deprived. By now, it was very smoky around our house, so my wife and I walked outside and around our property. No fires were visible. It's not unheard of for thick smoke to be blown into our area of Northern California from distant fires, so we didn't think too much of it. My shift started at 11:00 PM, and at 10:30 PM, I decided to head to work a little early.

When I arrived at the hospital, just two miles from my house, it seemed even smokier than it had been at my house. Early on, it was clear it was going to be an unusual shift; it was busy right away and I was seeing patients with smoke-related respiratory complaints and even a few who had been injured escaping fires in their homes. We were hearing about more and more fires in the area, and not long into the shift, a paramedic told me that "every fire asset in the county is deployed right now." That was the first time a chill ran up my back, and fear touched my brain. At the time of the fire, I was serving in the role of assistant physician-in-chief for hospital operations, and staff were beginning to approach me with concerns and complaints from patients as smoke intrusion into the hospital was becoming an issue. The surgeon on call paged me to ask if he should go forward with an appendectomy. As paramedics and firefighters brought us more and more patients, their radios chirped with traffic of various calls—structure fire here, grass fire there. Shortly before 1:00 AM on October 9, I heard one of those radio calls with an address that I figured could only be a few miles from our home. A quick Google search revealed it was, indeed, about three miles as the crow flies, so I called my wife and told her to get a few things together "just in case"—computers, wedding albums, and backup drives. Now it was just after 1:00 AM, and I had a patient in room twenty-four with an ankle injury (non-fire related). I was in the room with her and her friends showing her the x-ray of her ankle when my personal phone rang. It was my neighbor's name showing on my phone. It was 1:15 AM, just fifteen minutes since I had called my wife with the "just in case" warning. I apologized to the patient as I answered, and my neighbor yelled at me urgently: "Get out! Get out! Get out!" He didn't know I was at work, but I knew why he was yelling, and I said, "I have to go." I hung up and ran out of the room, immediately calling my wife again.

Only my daughter answered the phone. Screaming. Just screaming. What could I do? I had to help Sophie control her panic. Where was Claire? Panic.

Control your own breathing, Josh. Tell your daughter she's going to be okay. She's going to be okay, right? My colleague was wrapping up her shift and could hear Sophie screaming, could hear me trying to calm her, and immediately put down everything to call her husband and race home to evacuate her own family. Thirty to sixty seconds stretched on forever, but Claire's voice was suddenly there: "I'm in the car! We're driving! We're driving!" And then "We're down the hill!" "Just come to Kaiser" was all I could say.

About that time, my boss came to the emergency department. He had just fled his home surrounded by fire. The area manager and senior vice president, the on-call administrator phoned me: "Josh, what's going on? I'm getting calls about smoke in the hospital." "I think my house just burned down. I think we need to open the command center." She was on her way in, but not before flames were upon her in her home. By 1:30 AM, my wife and daughter were in the hospital. They were okay. They got the dogs out. Not the cat. Not the goats. Not the chickens. Not the snake. Not the fish.

Shortly after 2:00 AM, with the hospital command center operational, I received a call: "Josh, we need you in the command center." In addition to my work in the emergency department, I have traveled domestically and internationally to provide disaster relief work, and now my skills and experience were being called upon at home, something I never really imagined. My family was safe. I had work to do. They were going to head to the South Bay to stay with my wife's parents. I took on the role of "incident commander." Initially, we were in "surge mode," gearing up to accept more patients. However, at 3:30 AM, the fire incident commander came into our command center to utter another phrase I will always remember: "We're making our last stand." He outlined his plan to try to hold off the fire that was now burning through a mobile home park immediately adjacent to the hospital grounds. I was faced with the decision to hope that they would be successful or initiate evacuation of 124 patients from the hospital and emergency department, including patients in the ICU, which placed patients at considerable risk. One way or another, I was going to live with my decision. "Time to go." I was very fortunate to have colleagues Dr. Kirk Pappas (my boss) and Judy Coffey, RN, in the command center to affirm that decision, but I was keenly aware of the burden of responsibility I had accepted and now felt so strongly. I often encourage my pediatric patients by telling them that the definition of courage is not the absence of fear, but rather moving forward in the face of fear. It was around that time that I wondered to myself if all of Santa Rosa would burn down that night. I certainly felt fear.

By 6:30 AM, the hospital was safely empty of patients. An orange sun was rising through the unbelievably thick smoke. I was spent. The adrenaline was wearing off. When Claire and Sophie had been with me earlier that morning, Claire had described the fire driven by that angry wind swirling around her and the house, the trees exploding in flames, and the fire racing across the property. I had asked: "Did you actually see the house on fire?" "I'm pretty sure," she said.

So, I held on to hope. Maybe the house hadn't burned. Maybe somehow the cat had survived. I tried to get up to the house that afternoon, but there were downed power lines, and I couldn't be sure they were safe to cross. The whole scene looked apocalyptic, as if a huge bomb had gone off. Fires were still burning. There were smoldering shells of cars, and chimneys stood as tombstone markers where houses had once stood. Many times, I had been to disasters. I always knew that my time there would be limited, that eventually I would be going home to my bed. This time, I was not so sure I had a home or a bed to which I could return.

I made it back the next day. The entire neighborhood was obliterated. Hundreds of homes. As I turned up our hill, one lone house stood—our neighbors'—situated down the hill from us. I held out hope. I held my breath. I continued up the hill and around the corner. Not unexpectedly, but still absolutely stunningly, our home, all our belongings, and everything that held memories for me and marked my time on earth were laid to waste. Nothing but ash and smoldering wreckage. I jumped out of the car and called for the cat. I was gut punched and started to cry. I kept calling for the cat. I pleaded. He never came.

There was a happy moment, however. After a few minutes, over my calls came some bleating. Our two goats, Lucy and Ethel, emerged. Singed, but seemingly healthy, somehow miraculously having survived. To this day, we really don't know how. We imagine they huddled on a patch of dirt, the fire flashed through the grass and over them, and then burned their fence down but spared them. I also imagine my red-tail boa constrictor, a pet for twenty years, caught in his tank, writhing against the glass as our house caught flames and heated unbearably. And most painfully for me, I imagine our cat, frightened, confused, diving under our bed. My wife tried to run back in to find him. The power was out. Her retinas had the red flames of the fire burned in and it was hopeless. That was when I called, while she had tried desperately to find him. It's only a damn cat, but for me, that loss embodies my tenuous grip on things that are meaningful to me. Imagining his painful death, I am still overwhelmed, feeling that I let him down. What if I had been home? This is an enduring loss.

Going through medical school and residency, and then more than twenty years of practice, we witness pain and loss all the time; in some ways, it is our job to bear witness and validate. No doubt, I have had many opportunities to save a life or to reassure a patient and their family that they are going to be just fine, and they are grateful for the interaction. But for me, the most poignant, yet satisfying, patient interactions have been around death. I still remember the first patient whom I watched take his last breath as I sat with his wife and son when I was a third-year medical student. I remember the patient. He collapsed playing golf with his best friend who was visiting from the East Coast. As we scrambled to get him to a center where they might be able to intervene on his massive aortic dissection, I called his wife and best friend to the bedside before I intubated him. They got to say goodbye, and he died as he was being loaded onto a helicopter. And I still keep the letter written to me by the wife of a patient whom I diagnosed with advanced cancer who died a few weeks later. I took the time to have a very frank conversation with them and they wrote to tell me how important that was for them. We spoke about how much they had always loved dancing together over the years, and they made sure they could dance together a few more times.

But how do I have that conversation with myself? I was feeling guilty three days after the fire when I stopped at a light and told a homeless person asking for handouts, "Sorry, I have nothing, I lost it all in the fire." That was crazy. I was driving my nice car. I had a job and a bank account. He truly had nothing. And I continued to face that guilt: we were all okay. "We aren't dodging bullets or bombs. Why should I complain about our loss?" I said to a friend. He reminded me that I was setting an absurdly high bar.

I definitely felt adrift. My anchor was my past, and now all evidence of my past was gone. I drove faster. I sped around curves. I don't drink much, but I drank more. Why should I stay with my job? My marriage? Why should I bother building anything up when it can just be snatched away and burned to ash?

Claire and Sophie did get our two dogs out that night, Terra and Pete. But Pete suffered, too. He seemed more anxious, and all those moves did not help. He became more territorial and aggressive. At our old house, we had property, and no people or dogs walked past. He only saw other dogs and people when we were out walking. Now we were in a neighborhood with people and dogs walking past our home—his territory—every day, and he was getting more difficult to manage. One evening while Claire and I were out, Sophie was home with the dogs and a neighbor walked past. Pete managed to get the front door open and bolt outside, attacking the neighbor's dog. After paying some vet bills, the dog was okay, but we couldn't risk the possibility that the next time might be a child walking his puppy. Another dagger in my heart as I held a healthy dog being put down. Someone else I let down.

I feel okay these days. I know how lucky we are. My wife is steadfast and so passionate about our family. She says we're "fire survivors," not "fire victims," and she means it. Throughout this ordeal, I've had a good job, decent insurance, and a path forward. Building (or rebuilding) a house is very stressful and has gone on much longer than I ever imagined it would, but finally the end is in sight. Last year, I stepped away from my administrative role I held for twenty years. I started as assistant chief of the emergency department, then chief for eleven years, chair of the ED chiefs of Kaiser Permanente Northern California (twenty-one departments), and finally assistant physician-in-chief. I gave up some salary, bonuses, and prestige because the reality we learned is what we have is right here, right now. We put off trips and events "until next year," but now I've come to realize that next year might not ever come. We all know this on some level, but when you lose virtually everything you've ever had, the perspective becomes different and you give more than just lip service to the concept. While I'm a naturally optimistic person, a portion of my optimism was carved out on October 9. Every day, every interaction shapes us incrementally, imperceptibly. That day was a cataclysmic shift, and I will remember always what I lost, never to regain. So, I want to make sure I take the time for a few more dances with my wife.

Joshua Weil, M.D.
Emergency Medicine

DESPERATE FOR DAWN

Blown by the wind
Calm after the storm
Powered by the sun
Bullied by the moon
The undulating sea
Spawns relentless variation

While a rising tide
Gently rids the sand of any recollection

Warren R. Dunn
University of South Florida College of Medicine
Class of 1997

SURRENDER

The insects of imagination
Bug my brain and crawl in my veins
Centuries of mutation
Laughing at my humiliation
The weight of this twisted ladder on my back
Climbing the rungs of regret
Trying to repair, fix, and heal what is broken
A recovery laden with so much pain
Healed or cured is hard to claim
A cardinal number four, this boy
Defying the hedonic hunt for a better toy
Beholden to the patient soul
Behind those beautiful green eyes
That no longer bear the burden of disease
Surrender all hope of a different past
Let go
Feel the forgiving pull of gravity
Dance in the collective unconscious clouds
Of an otherwise crystal-clear torment from long ago

Warren R. Dunn, M.D.
Orthopedic Surgery

THE RIGHT PROFESSION

"Dr. Manson, there is a first-year medical student in my office who will be working with you this week. Can you come over now? Thanks." The secretary smiled at me sweetly. "He'll be right over," she said. "Have a seat."

As I nervously waited, I tried to picture Dr. Manson, whom I was to follow for part of my summer clerkship. This was my first time to work in a hospital and with a "real" doctor. I pictured Dr. Manson as a cross between my grandfather and Billy Graham. The image seemed to fit his name. I was startled out of my reverie when a young man, not much older than myself, walked in. "Dr. Manson," the secretary began her introductions. Ah yes, I had forgotten about the "hierarchy of medicine." No medical student ever works directly with an attending physician. This work is reserved for the residents. "Poor Resident Manson. He must be the newest of them all to get stuck with me," I thought.

For this week, my job was to be his shadow. His job was to let me follow. He was under no obligation to necessarily explain things to me. He didn't even have to speak to me if he didn't want to. As my first day wore on, my nervousness gave way to relief. I found Dr. Manson to be a kind and willing teacher. He also treated me with respect, introducing me as "Doctor" when we met new patients. I later found this was not the norm with students.

We were on a general internal medicine rotation. There were three different teams, and I was placed on the "A-Team." Although there was no best team, I couldn't help but smile to myself at that name. I began to imagine our team saving lives daily and bringing patients safely away from the face of death—just like Trapper John, M.D. Soon I learned how skewed my thinking was. I also learned that saving patients from death is sometimes the last thing one wants to do.

It seemed to be a week for strokes. The word *stroke* is a general term for what is usually a spontaneous loss of blood to part of the brain. Often, this is called a cerebrovascular event or, perhaps more appropriately, a cerebrovascular accident. This can be caused by many things, including a blow to the head and subsequent blood clot (hematoma); a clot in a blood vessel supplying the brain, which keeps oxygen from reaching part of the brain (ischemia); or a blood vessel bursting and leaking blood into the brain (hemorrhage). Strokes are, I learned, one of the leading causes of death in our country.

Lily was her name. She was my first stroke patient. Having suffered a clot in her middle cerebral artery, a major vessel to the brain, her prognosis was not good. The part of her brain responsible for speech (Broca's area) was destroyed from lack of oxygen. However, the area in her brain that allowed her to understand speech and symbols (Wernicke's area) was intact. How very frustrating it must have been to understand and yet not be able to respond. In addition, she was hemiplegic (paralyzed on one side of her body). She was what one doctor called a "typical stroke patient." I was told to compare her reflexes on her normal side to the ones on the side that was paralyzed, as they would be noticeably different. She was able to squeeze fingers on command with her normal hand. Although there was facial weakness, she was able to move her eyes fairly well while following a moving object.

One night, I took a fellow student, Alan, up to the hospital while I checked on my team's patients. When we got to Lily's room, we talked to her some and I showed him the interesting parts of her examination. I noticed her eyes were moving a little better and told her so. I asked Alan to let her grab his fingers. Then I asked her to squeeze my fingers too. Lily still could not move one hand. We had asked her to perform this action many times, looking for improvement and had yet to find any. This time though, she did not let go of my fingers, but held them tightly in her strong hand. I looked up at her eyes—one had secretions all around it due to lack of enervation of that side of her face. Her eye that was normally dry, however, now had tears rolling out of it and down her face. I held back tears of my own as I tried to reassure her. There had been a note from her family leaving details of their next time to visit. I relayed this to her as well, giving her the biggest smile I could muster. Soon, we moved on to the other patients. When I lay down that night, though, I thought of her—and then said my prayers. I wondered if I could learn to deal with this sadness I felt on a daily basis for Lily and others. I wondered if I had chosen the right profession.

One morning, I came in and Dr. Manson told me we had another patient with a possible stroke. "Oh, no," I thought. "I don't know if I can get used to this." He must have seen my saddened expression because he quickly went on to explain that this man had most likely experienced a TIA. "What's that?" I asked.

"It stands for transient ischemic attack. It's like a small stroke where the brain loses a tiny part of its oxygen supply for a short time and then quickly recovers." I opened my pocketbook, *Care of the Medical Patient*, and read up on TIAs. Patients usually experience an episode of weakness or even paralysis generally associated with confusion. Normally, permanent damage does not occur. Hopefully, this would be the case with Mr. Atkinson.

When Dr. Manson and I went in to examine Mr. Atkinson, we found him to be confused and weak on one side of his body. He was able to remember some things though, which gave everyone hope. Dr. Manson performed a lumbar puncture in his lower back to draw out some of his cerebrospinal fluid surrounding the spinal cord. This was done to rule out meningitis as a cause for his confusion. This procedure was very necessary but also very painful. I assisted Dr. Manson by holding the patient in a fetal position on his side. His daughter was there and helped too. She cried softly, and I knew it was painful for her to see her father this way.

Luckily, his story had a happy ending. The test for meningitis was negative. On examination a few days later, he was completely oriented and was gaining strength in his weak side. Dr. Manson and I both came out of the room smiling. No words were necessary. We both knew now that he would be fine.

In a few days, it was time for Mr. Atkinson to leave the hospital. Dr. Manson and I went to say goodbye. I was sad to see him go. He was a happy case on a ward of many sad ones. We left his room and headed toward the cafeteria for lunch, talking about medicine. The entire week, I had been feeling lost in a sea of terminology and diseases I knew nothing about. "There's so much I don't know," I finally confessed. "How will I ever learn it all?" There, I had said it—one of my greatest fears that seemed so overwhelming. Dr. Manson was so knowledgeable and confident in his work; yet he replied, "There's still so much I don't even know." He smiled. "That's the way it is with medicine. There's always more, and you always do your very best with what you know."

Just then, Mr. Atkinson's daughter ran up behind us. "Oh, I'm so glad I caught you. I missed your goodbye earlier in my father's room, but I did want to thank you both for all you did for him. You all were wonderful!" Then she shook Dr. Manson's hand. As I held mine out, she grabbed it and pulled me into a hug. Then she was gone. "How grateful she is," I thought, "and how little we actually did." Yet suddenly in that moment, the mass of knowledge I was so worried about acquiring did not seem too large anymore. The memory of her smile and gratitude had me on a cloud all day. I knew I had chosen the right profession.

Stephanie P. Swafford
Texas A&M University College of Medicine
Class of 1997

THE RIGHT PROFESSION— PART II

There is no doubt in my mind, now twenty-five years after being a medical student, that I have chosen the right profession. Having been an ob/gyn for most of my career, I continually feel blessed with the work I get to do each and every day. Truly, what a privilege it is to be a part of people's most joyful and lifechanging events. Obstetrics is a unique field, allowing for close relationships, not only with patients, but their families as well. It was such an honor to participate in so many special birth moments of patients I had grown to know and love.

However, it is the counterbalance of the joy that should have been that causes tragedy to cut so deep when things don't go well. It never gets easier to explain that the baby they are carrying is no longer alive. The anxiety of a difficult delivery does not quickly diminish. The fatigue of many sleepless nights takes its toll—usually on my own family and children. Yet, through all the struggles they have heard me walk through and all the missed ball games and recitals, my own children remain understanding and proud that the patients they will never meet have been cared for so well. And, they have shared graciously.

It is also wonderful to see so many patients each day for annual exams that I have known for over two decades. I love seeing teenagers and children, young women, menopausal women, and those near the end of life. It is such a blessing to know women on such a deep level. There are many I have shared their greatest joys and deepest sorrows. I have walked with many women, not only through the births of their children, but also the infidelity of their spouses, the death of their husbands and children, and the diagnosis of cancer. The discomfort of giving a difficult diagnosis never gets easier, but the joys of survival and recovery are all the sweeter for the painful road that was embarked upon.

Perhaps the most surprising blessing of all is that I have learned so much from my patients as well. Through the sharing of their lives, the wisdom they've imparted, and the health maintenance they have modeled, I have personally learned much and shared my learnings with other patients. They have shown me the power of faith and positive thinking when facing a mountain to climb. They have also shown me the power of love and how to die gracefully.

Yes, I can think of no better profession than being a physician. Through touching others, our lives are touched as well. True, the road is rough . . . but also richly rewarding.

Stephanie Swafford Bruce, M.D.
Obstetrics & Gynecology

TELEGRAM FROM ANOTHER PLANET

Dear Mom and Dad,

I'm sorry it's taken me so long to answer your last letter. I am in survival mode. I work from 6 AM until 7 PM every day of the week, except Sunday, and I have all-night call every third night. If I sleep on call nights, it is for two hours on the floor of the surgery floor conference room. If call night falls on a Sunday, I work all of Sunday too. I am on the trauma team, and I have lost count of the number of young men I have watched die in the last three weeks. At first, I kept track of them: the seventeen-year-old who jumped off a cliff, the drug dealer shot through the heart, the twenty-three-year-old who wrapped his sports car around a tree and had a love letter on a wrinkled piece of notebook paper in his pocket, and the unhelmeted motorcyclist who left his brain on the sidewalk. Now they are starting to blend into one archetypal young man with a handsome face and beautiful broken body; a crushed skull and an opened chest; tubes in his mouth, nose, groin, arms, and sides; and a bracelet around his ankle that reads, "Unidentified Black Male/900 27 48."

In the operating room, I see the face of God. The opalescent lights, the beeping of all the monitors, and the glint of the instruments put me into a trance. The glory of creation in the pulsing of blood vessels and the pattern of sinews brings on a feeling like ecstasy. I run home and scrawl with lipstick on my bathroom mirror: "I LOVE SURGERY! ! !" My closest friend on the service will barely speak to me anymore because, he says, I act like a jock. "I like the other Jan," he says. There is no other Jan. This is just Jan adapting to the current situation. I feel as though I am being flayed alive of all the soft appurtenances of civilized humanity, and what is left is lean and strong and hard with a dull shine like gunmetal. This is Jan who rowed lightweight for Radcliffe crew and trained cross country so hard she stress-fractured her fibula at seventeen. This is Jan who rode a motorcycle in the Peace Corps, carried dead babies back to their mothers, knelt in pools of blood on the highway, went without food for three days, and swam to the island in the bay. I laugh loudly at coarse jokes about the two suicide attempts we operated on earlier in the week. One guy washed down twenty-five Demerol with a cup each of Clorox and ammonia; when this modern version of a hemlock cocktail failed to kill him, he stabbed himself several times in the chest, then slashed his throat. My chief resident ligated his jugular veins and let me staple his neck back together. His head was held on with staples; he looks like an inner-city Frankenstein. The other guy stabbed himself in the belly. He refused to cooperate with anyone in the ER and was generally such a pain that, though his peritoneal lavage was equivocally normal, the residents did an exploratory laparotomy on him just to shut him up and teach him a lesson. We put the would-be suicides in the same room on the surgery floor so they could compare notes about methods for next time.

I have reverted to a creature of the jungle. I forage among the trays of food left by patients for cellophane-wrapped slices of bread, pints of milk and orange juice, graham crackers, packets of saltines, and little trays of peanut butter and jelly. I eat at 3 AM on the elevator from the sixth floor to the emergency room if it's a modified trauma; if it's a major trauma, I run down the stairs while gulping down a carton of milk. In this way, I keep all of my 125 pounds on my frame, while my friend on the service has lost weight standing through eight-hour surgeries and missing meals. I find corners in which to sleep between emergencies and surgeries: ten minutes, twenty minutes, an hour, before my beeper or my watch goes off. I steal pillows from empty patient rooms to make my bed on the floor; I lift blankets from laundry carts and pinch tiny toothpaste tubes from supply cabinets. I have labs to look up and patients to examine and charts to write in before 7 AM rounds. I ignore the man on the stretcher behind me addressing me as "Nurse" and asking for a cup of water. In hell, I would dip my finger in the water to wet the lips of Lazarus in torment, but in the hospital, I am much too busy.

The other day, I fainted in the OR. I've never fainted before in my life. It was quite an experience. It was not from being grossed out by anything—I have an unbelievably high gross-out threshold. In fact, the only thing I can think of that grossed me out in recent memory is when a guy I knew named Peter had a girlfriend who had his baby, and afterward Peter fried up the placenta with onions and tried to get his girlfriend to eat it with him: "For the vitamins." The morning I fainted, I was merely watching a routine hernia repair, of which I'd already seen several. It was not disgust but exhaustion and terror that caused me to go pale and clammy. The surgeon was an extremely talented teacher who strove mightily to overcome his natural antipathy toward women. That day, he was failing. He was "pimping" me, asking me questions, and I didn't seem to have any of the right answers. Everything I did was wrong, and he was calling me "sister" in that special tone that men like him reserve for people without Y chromosomes, when I just said, "Doctor M., I feel ill," handed him my retractor, stepped back against the wall, and slid gently to the floor. I never actually lost consciousness, but let us say that consciousness was briefly and radically altered. I couldn't keep my eyes open, and though I could hear the voices of the surgeons and nurses, it was like listening from the bottom of a well. I knew that the "she" they were mentioning must be me, but I didn't quite identify with whomever they were talking about. I was loaded onto a stretcher by the anesthesiologists and wheeled down the hall to a holding area, where I took advantage of my first opportunity to lie still with my eyes closed in something like thirty hours. Fifteen minutes later, I was back in the OR, but I wasn't allowed to scrub in— "Why don't you just watch for a while?" Guess I'm just not The Right Stuff.

This is why I have not had time to write. This is why, when I tell you that I miss you, that I send you my love, that I am happy for Johnny and Heidi expecting their baby, and that I am glad for David and Maggie and congratulate them on their engagement, I feel as though I am sending you a telegram from another planet.

Love,
Jan

Jan Steckel
Yale University School of Medicine
Class of 1994

YOU CAN SCRUB OUT
ANY TIME YOU LIKE, BUT
YOU CAN NEVER LEAVE

Call it burnout, posttraumatic stress disorder, depression, or anxiety. As a pediatrician in training at The Children's Hospital in Boston, I had it. During the second half of my internship, I kept a large syringe, tubing, and a butterfly needle under some clothing in my bottom dresser drawer. I was afraid of making a medical mistake that would lead to the death of one of my child patients, and I didn't think I could handle it if I did. My plan was that if that happened, I would kill myself with an air embolism.

As sleep deprivation and the humiliations of ritual hazing accumulated, my emotional condition got worse. Many mornings when I woke up, I wished I could kill myself before I had to go into work at the hospital. I thought about jumping off a bridge into the Charles River. One early spring, when I was an undergraduate, a friend of mine had found the body of a woman in the Charles while he was out sculling. She had apparently been trapped in the ice over the winter and been freed to float in the thaw. The closest bridge to me, though, was a half-hour walk away. By the time I got there, I would be late to work, and I couldn't stand being late. So, I went to work instead, which felt more or less like hitting concrete headfirst at terminal velocity anyway.

Luckily for me, I got out of the practice of medicine before I ever killed anyone by accident. Many physicians do, though, some time in their careers. I remember my senior resident in pediatrics telling me when I was an intern that we pediatricians couldn't make mistakes like other doctors because it was not permissible to cause a child's death. Maybe that kind of thinking was why a senior resident at a hospital near mine took his own life while I was a resident. He had a nurse put an IV in his arm, ostensibly for antibiotics, then went home and injected himself with potassium chloride.

As a retired physician for twenty years, I still have nightmares in which I'm a doctor again. Usually in these dreams, I have done or am doing an internal medicine residency in addition to the pediatrics residency I actually completed. Often, the adult residency is at Mass General, also in Boston, where my father was doing his own internship when I was born.

I spend a considerable amount of my time these days taking phone calls and emails from friends and family who want medical advice. I always tell them that I can't give it to them, as I long ago let my medical license lapse and am no longer a doctor. In any case, I am a retired baby doc, not a physician for adults. That never fazes them, so I go so far as to explain to them medical terminology on their lab report that they don't understand or tell them whether I think they ought to call their physicians or go to an emergency room for their current emergency. It never fails to amaze me that people who have private or managed-care primary care doctors don't realize that they can call an on-call doctor for their practice, even when their own doctor is not in the office. So, I explain that again, and again. I walk them through the healthcare system, tell them how to request home care or a social work consult, or how to get their questions answered, just not by me.

Several of them have asked me to be the designated proxy on their advance healthcare directives. I have helped manage end-of-life care for a few people that way. It is a huge burden that reactivates what I call my PTSD (though I have never been formally diagnosed with that disorder), and I have developed a higher threshold for saying, "Yes."

My father and his father were physicians, but my mother was a psychiatric social worker. I seem to have combined the roles. When I became disabled by chronic pain and couldn't drive or go out much, many of the friends who stuck with me and were willing to visit me at home were older people who had empathy for my physical limitations. Over the last decade, they've started to die, and I find myself assisting their families, or for those who don't have close surviving relatives, communicating their wishes to their doctors and the progress of their final decline to their friends. It is exhausting, and it is a role I am more than ready to give up.

Since I started reading in January 2020 about a new viral pneumonia that was killing people in the Wuhan province of China, I've been having the doctor nightmares more frequently. I could see the COVID-19 pandemic coming and tried to warn my relatives, friends, and neighbors about it. I told them to make sure they had working thermometers and Tylenol or Advil in their houses. I said they should buy a few extra nonperishables each time they shopped and slowly build up a couple weeks' worth of food in case they had to self-quarantine or shelter in place. I told my cousins that when their elderly parents were eventually stuck sheltering at home, they should develop a phone and email rotation of who would check on them each day to make sure that they were okay and that they didn't get too lonely. Some people listened, but others thought I was hysterical. My home health aide told me I was decreasing the vibration of the world by spreading fear and causing the pandemic to manifest by dwelling on the possibility.

My home health aide, cleaning lady, and gardener all stopped coming when the San Francisco Bay Area locked down in the middle of March. The gardener returned in July, but case numbers are going up again in California, so I don't know how long she'll want to keep coming. I am delighted that the cleaning lady got her BA and is going on to better work. The home health aide, who did all my errands and some of my cooking and who drove me places for a decade, started posting so many conspiracy theories about the pandemic and antivaccination propaganda memes on her Facebook page that I don't think I can have her back to work again. I'm high risk for COVID-19 in four different ways and can't have someone in my home who's not willing to get an influenza shot in the fall. One of my close relatives contracted COVID-19 during the pandemic and later had a psychotic episode. A couple of older, chronically ill poetry friends died.

I was a very prolific writer, but since the COVID-19 pandemic started six months ago, I've only written two poems. One was published immediately; the other was so bad I never sent it out. They were both pandemic poems. I don't know whether I'm not writing because I'm so horrified by our government's failure to protect us from the disease, or if I'm just exhausted from all the extra housework, yard work, cooking, laundry, disinfecting, ordering by delivery, handling of packages, and emotional care of relatives and friends. I seem to work nonstop on all of that and my medical editing from dawn to dusk, leaving no time or energy for creativity. This is the first piece of creative nonfiction I've written in half a year. I'm so appalled by the state of our country that I'm nearly speechless.

Since March, no one has entered our house except my husband and me. Half a dozen people have had dinner in our backyard in ones or twos, six to eight feet away from us. I do this about once a week. I wear a mask and gloves when I prepare and serve their food and only take them off when I sit down to eat a safe distance away from them. I don't want to spread anything to anybody. I've gone for a few socially distanced walks with friends and relatives, but people seem to have a hard time maintaining a six-foot distance from me when they're walking and talking, so I do most of my walking by myself or with my husband. I can't do it in my own neighborhood because most people don't socially distance or wear masks here. I go to the richer neighborhoods, where people have the privilege to work at home, don't live eight people to a two-bedroom apartment, and have enough leisure time to read and watch lots of news. Most of those people wear masks and stay six feet away from me, though not all.

Because I worked in operating rooms and in research labs, I have a good grasp of sterile techniques. That has combined with a few thousand years of kosher/housewife genes to make me, as my niece says, more "diligent" than most people about precautions during the pandemic. I also feel quite vulnerable because of my various health conditions. I hope I'm not developing obsessive-compulsive disorder or being way more careful than is good for me. I try to get out of the house on most days so that I don't develop agoraphobia, but I'll admit it: being around people other than my husband these days makes me nervous.

The other night, I had two relatives over to eat in the backyard with my husband and me. Instead of playing charades after dinner, we took the Beck Depression Inventory. Three out of the four of us had mildly depressed mood, though no clinical depression. I didn't really appreciate until I took the test how sad I had been feeling. I wonder when or if I will feel the need to reach out to a mental healthcare professional about my mood. It seems like the appropriate response to the situation, and not too severe. Many of my friends and relatives are similarly a bit downcast.

I sometimes try to tell people that I expect the fall and winter to get a lot worse. I describe what flu season was like for me when I was a pediatrician and might see forty patients in a three-hour evening clinic. I say that influenza strains our medical system every year as it is and that COVID-19 on top of that is almost certain to overwhelm our capacity. A particularly virulent flu season could mean catastrophe. I ask people to get their flu shots early. I wonder how we're going to continue to get together outside when it's cold and raining, whether COVID-19 rates will go up as a result of being together more inside, and what more isolation and sickness will do to our morale. I remember how hard it was for me to get certain provisions delivered to my home, especially paper products and disinfectants, during the first peak. Grocery deliveries became delayed for up to a week, and then I'd only get half of what I ordered. As a result, I've filled my garage with supplies for the next peak.

Among those supplies are extra acetaminophen, ibuprofen, gloves, shower caps, masks, an extra thermometer with disposable sleeves, a pulse oximeter, face shields, and an old surgical gown for visiting sick neighbors or caring for my relatives if the healthcare system gets overwhelmed. There are even adult diapers and disposable underpads for my husband and me to care for each other if one of us is too weak or dizzy to get up to use the bathroom. I remember when I used to set up my code carts or my instrument trays in advance so that I wouldn't have to scramble for medicines or tools at the last minute. I felt as a doctor, and I still feel today, that if I think everything through in advance and am prepared for the worst possibilities, that I am safer and that others around me are safer too. My New Age acquaintances might say I am bringing the worst into existence by thinking about it and giving it energy, but that's not how my mind works. My mind, two decades after I left medical practice, works like a doctor's. So, I practice in my nightmares, and I hope I won't need to use my knowledge or my supplies. I don't want to be a doctor again.

Jan Steckel, M.D.
Pediatrics

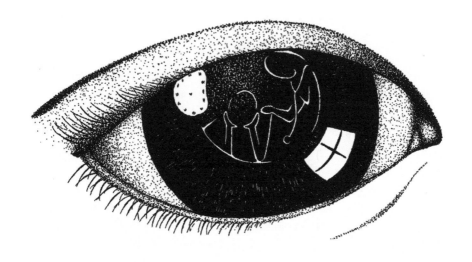

20/20
Then - ink

Sue Rhee
Albany Medical College
Class of 1998

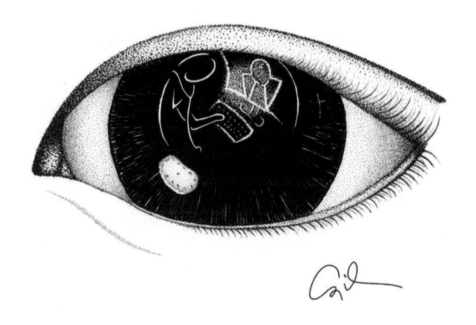

20/20
Now - iPencil

Sue Rhee, M.D.
Pediatrics & Gastroenterology

After the Storm

The first thing she saw was white.
The lights.
Then the ceiling.
One, then the other, one, then the other.
She was dizzy from the pace.
And then she stopped. Abruptly.
The coats. The white coats.
One, then two, then three, four.
A tornado of movement swirled around her.
Beads of rain sizzled on her naked skin.
Thunder beat hard on her chest, and the pain, the pain.
She was drowning in the pain rising like a flood from her feet to her knees,
her chest. She gasped.
Her eyes.
Fluttering glimpses of white and she whispered,
"God, let it be o . . ."
"Very carefully, so as not to damage superficial nerves,
    make an incision from the jugular notch to the xiphisternal junction."
The first thing I cut was skin.
The flesh.
Then muscle.
Separating one from the other. Flesh from muscle.
    I was dizzy from the smell.
    And then I stopped.
    The face. I stopped to look at the face.
"One, two, three, four," I counted, and then removed the white cloth.
    And saw the aftermath of a wretched storm.

80

Blackness filled the sockets that had seen herself alive.
As I see myself.
A face that had drowned in the pain of wanting to live.
Like I live.
My mind.
Fluttering glimpses of her life.
And my life.
And how each has made the other understand.

Leanne Marie Yanni
State University of New York Health Science Center at Syracuse
College of Medicine
Class of 1998

EACH HAS MADE THE OTHER UNDERSTAND

Each has made the other understand. That line from a poem I wrote over twenty years ago foreshadowed a theme that has evolved over the course of my career. When my children were little, I read books to them called *ValueTales*. Each told a famous individual's story and the value it exemplified, such as compassion, courage, and humility. Below I share several stories, each representing a complex lesson that has shaped me into the physician I continue to become.

Woodrow Wilson was not a president. He was a patient I cared for in the early years of my career. Month after month, when he came to see me, it was the same routine. Looking over his reading glasses, he would lower his newspaper as I entered the room and say, "Doc, how are you?" Then, as I left the room, he would say, "Doc, take care of yourself." He developed idiopathic pulmonary fibrosis, a terminal diagnosis. Shortly before his death, he was admitted to the hospital. I sat on the side of his bed, his untouched morning newspaper folded beside him with his reading glasses as a paperweight. He said he was grateful. As I stood up to leave, he called to me one last time, "Doc, take care of yourself." I hear his voice often, especially when work has led me to exhaustion or when faced with a dissonant choice. First take care of yourself, he taught me, or you will not have the strength to compassionately care for others.

Eleanor was the mother of a respected colleague with more years of internal medicine experience than I had been alive. When that colleague asked me to care for his mother who was in declining health, I had said, "Of course," though I had felt some trepidation—mostly fear of making a mistake. Eleanor was in her nineties with severe aortic stenosis and was intelligent enough to refuse interventions that would likely have hastened her death. The classic stairstep functional decline was ensuing; after several office visits, I instinctively asked, "Why don't I come see you at home?" I counted the many steps that climbed to the front door of her hillside home. On my arrival, Eleanor was lying comfortably in bed beneath a quilt her grandmother had made. This would prove to be a precious last visit with her; she died peacefully in her own home—a wish she had shared with me. My colleague had entrusted me with the care of his mother; his confidence in me superseded the confidence I had in myself, and I had climbed the stairs he set before me.

Fernando was an athlete and a father, my age at the time, with meta-static colon cancer. The discussion we had about the benefit and burden of nephrostomy tubes when his kidneys failed has not been surpassed as *the* most difficult conversation of my career. He chose several more months of life by placing the tubes, despite a high probability of severe pain as the cancer grew; dying naturally of kidney failure is the body's safeguard to prevent an unimaginable level of suffering as cancer spreads to the pelvic organs and spinal nerves. We tried every available medication; the pain would abate for a short time, but then rage again. Finally, I put him in the hospital and begged the anesthesiologist to place an epidural catheter to deliver pain medication directly into the spine. "It won't last," the anesthesiologist said, "Why do it?" I was courageously insistent: "He is screaming in pain and this will be a memory his family will not forget." He understood and placed the catheter. Finally, Fernando experienced peace. However, I saw the life leaving his pale and sunken eyes. His wife, kneeling at his bedside, needed to be told. With difficulty, I summoned the words, "He is dying," and spoke them aloud. Almost immediately, his entire family surrounded his bedside. The light streaming in from the hospital window formed a halo around them. They held his body as life left him. "God—give them courage," I prayed, "like you gave me."

Kim was only a teenager. She suffered with Ehlers-Danlos syndrome and all its complications—no longer able to eat, no longer able to sit up, in constant pain. She required daily intravenous nutrients and medications on an intricate schedule. The room was always cool and dark; both temperature and lighting were adjusted to help manage her most severe symptoms. Light shown through a high window illuminated the stuffed animals strewn around the upper perimeters of the living room, now a permanent bedroom. A new doctor was challenging for them; the mother–daughter team had to reexplain and renegotiate treatment regimens designed through years of trial and error. Over months, I thought, "I can't go there again; I offer, and they decline; I explain, and they refute; I adjust, and they revert." I was determined not to give up though. Eventually, it became easier. Through patience and humility, I found Kim was generally right about her body's response to medications and other interventions. It was I who needed to listen and learn. As a physician, we need to not always be in control; letting go of this illusion was another step toward professional maturity.

Joel admitted himself to the hospital for pain and dehydration, though he wasn't going to die any time soon. The oncologist and I agreed on this: localized pancreatic cancer; it would be months at least, possibly more than a year. He was Jewish, of deep faith, and believed God was ready for him. He called his daughter home from Israel and summoned his rabbi. It was one of the few times in my palliative care career that the patient's assessment of prognosis was shorter than the physician's. Despite improvement in his symptoms, he continued to have faith in his own impending death. Though scientifically implausible, God called for him right on cue. A physician need not be scientifically certain in these matters; what we should be most certain about is our own uncertainty. For Joel, this was faith.

My career to date has been like a series of *ValueTales* titled "Care of Self," "Confidence," "Courage," "Letting Go," and "Faith." I could not have anticipated these gifts, but each gift has helped me understand more deeply and carry that understanding forward to others; and just as was foreshadowed at the start of my career with a patient who painfully gave life to my own learning, *Each has made the other understand.*

Leanne Yanni, M.D.
Internal Medicine & Palliative Medicine

Long, Long Ago

"Can I play another song for you, Grandpop?"

"Toselli's Serenade, sweetie."

In the white-walled kitchen, I remember you singing opera, gray-haired ponytail, like a samurai from my sculpting with water.

You and I alone in this little concert hall, telling me louder, louder, crescendo! Sing!

Coffee still on the table and the others in the living room, but here you stayed, a private audience for a little girl playing a violin.

"Long, Long Ago," you'd request, and sing along with great emotion. And sometimes cry. Now I wonder what in that song made you weep.

As you were dying, Grandpop, in the white-walled hospital room, I played for you, a private concert.

"Can I play another song for you, Grandpop?"

And the last words you said were "more music."

Mary C. Rorro
University of Medicine and Dentistry of New Jersey
School of Osteopathic Medicine
Class of 1995

THE GREATEST GIFT

"The music in my heart I bore, Long after it was heard no more."
—William Wordsworth

When I was six-and-a-half years old, my mother showed me her three-quarter-size violin that she used to play as a young girl. "I'm so proud that I can give this violin to you, Mary. You will love to play it as much as I did," she said. I cherished that violin and toted it about in its diminutive case. My parents enrolled me in Suzuki classes at Westminster Choir College in Princeton. Every Saturday, the ritual was to awaken early, tune my instrument, and saw away with the best and brightest of Princeton's young Suzuki protégés.

My brother and I progressed through the various books of the popular Japanese learning method. We played along to Suzuki records with our mother standing by the record player in our living room.

A photographer from the local newspaper came to the house to photograph our mother–daughter duo, and we made the next day's paper. It is one of our treasured pictures, both of us beaming with our violins tucked under our chins, facing the camera, I in a long ponytail and white winter outfit, and she, a glamorous young mother with a brilliant smile.

One of my teachers from Westminster used to craft stories about the pieces to connect music to words and impart an inherent sense of the lyrical nature of the music. An enthusiastic listener told me once, "You really make that violin talk." In high school, I played viola in the Princeton University Orchestra and took lessons there and was principal violist in the Greater Princeton Youth Orchestra. Those experiences, in addition to attending

Interlochen, the National Orchestral Institute and New Jersey Governor's School of Arts, honed my skills and instilled appreciation of classical symphonic works and chamber music.

As a daughter of a doctor and with other family members who were physicians, I told my parents at four years old about my desire to become one as well to help people. They served as medical and professional role models. My father had a home office, and my aunt was one of four pioneering women doctors in her Hahnemann medical school class in the 1950s.

My grandfather used to sing opera accompanied by my violin to a melody called "Toselli's Serenade." He performed it with a deep, earnest delivery, full of emotion. He came from Italy as a young man and carried the music of his Italian ancestors in his soul.

A heartbreaking moment was playing Toselli's serenade for my grandfather as he was dying in his hospital bed, where his final words were "more music." I felt spiritually connected to my grandfather through music as he transitioned from one world to the next. He was ushered to Heaven with the music he cherished, and this musical memory stays with me always.

Music would accompany me throughout my life and would become an essential component to soothe patients. After seeing the impact music had upon my grandfather's passing, my mother took me to perform for patients as a candy striper volunteering at the hospital where I was born.

She witnessed a depressed cancer patient who had not spoken for weeks begin to sing along with my violin to Christmas carols. It was one of many steering musical moments that influenced me to pursue my desire to become a physician and blend music into my life and profession. My mother was so proud, and the adoring look in her eyes as the music played inspired me to help others through the healing arts of music and medicine.

Bryn Mawr College was an academic sanctuary on the Main Line of Philadelphia that supported their students in community engagement. As president and principal violinist of the Bryn Mawr-Haverford Orchestra, I arranged benefit concerts for children with AIDS. My teacher from the Philadelphia Orchestra, Bryn Mawr, and Haverford nurtured my musical talent, and I was the recipient of Bryn Mawr's first Performing Arts Prize.

In medical school, I developed programs called "Musical Rounds: The Next Best Thing to Grand Rounds" and "From Soup to Notes" to perform for those in soup kitchens. Engaging with my fellow students and professors as we played for patients during our musical rounds was a bonding experience for us and our patients. Patients saw providers in another perspective, sharing our time and talent with them.

In medical school, I initiated a rotation in performing arts medicine in Puglia at the University of Bari, Italy. Employing the healing arts to improve patients' lives was an initiative I vowed to continue in my career.

Psychiatry was not my initial specialty choice. I planned to treat the medical problems of performing artists and was the student liaison of an organization called the International Arts Medicine Association. I was drawn to the mental health field during a psychiatry rotation at a state psychiatric hospital.

I was intrigued by my psychiatric supervisor's approach and the various patients in the ward. They came from all walks of life, and their moving stories—many dealing with trauma and loss—compelled me to help those with mental health issues.

I matched with a Harvard medical school psychiatry residency that placed me in the Veterans Administration (VA) system, as well as esteemed mental health hospitals, including McLean and Cambridge among others, and was chief resident of my program where I was named Chief Resident of the Year from the Pfizer Corporation in Washington, D.C.

During a Fellowship in Addiction Psychiatry at Massachusetts General Hospital, I was fortunate to have masterful mentors in an incredibly stimulating intellectual environment. It was an honor to interact and collaborate with Harvard physicians during residency and at MGH, which we then called "Man's Greatest Hospital." I was excited to walk up to the main doors, as there was new medical knowledge to absorb each day.

The visceral challenges and heartaches with which a physician is confronted with in medicine shaped my perspective on others and the world. Years of tests and training, long nights on call half-sleeping on starched sheets, are all worth it when someone says, "You changed my life."

I created a program in the VA called "A Few Good Notes," in which I play viola for veteran patients in their individual and group therapy sessions. Expanding it nationally through the VA system enables other employees to share music with veterans at their own VA hospitals.

Listening along with their buddies to selections of holiday, patriotic, and Broadway tunes, some veterans stand at attention and salute when the Marine Corps Hymn is played and grow quiet with "Silent Night." The music evokes memories and emotions, including one Vietnam vet who tearfully recalled that soldiers sang "Silent Night" on a hill in Vietnam, causing a ceasefire for that time on Christmas Eve. A patient recounted hearing a Bob Hope concert, but from a distance, as he was not allowed to attend the concert and had to stay out in the field. A World War II vet requested "I'll Be Seeing You in All the Old Familiar Places," as that was the last song he and his musician brother played before his brother drowned after his Navy destroyer was sunk by a torpedo. "I'll Be Home for Christmas" is difficult to hear for some veterans still burdened by survivor guilt. A veteran who stopped playing his guitar after returning from Vietnam was motivated to resume after hearing me play "Amazing Grace" in the office, saying his joy for the instrument came alive once more.

The Guitar Instruction Group (GIG) was initiated so veterans can learn and actively have music in their lives. Veterans teach other veterans guitar, and now they are music makers. The program has been "instrumental" in their treatment experience as a positive outlet for expression. We play together on viola and guitar, and one commented, "When you are here, Doc, you are one of us." A patient accompanied me to play guitar at Drumthwacket, the New Jersey Governor's mansion for the annual Marine Corps birthday ceremony, and at a presentation at St. Peter's University about the "A Few Good Notes" program. He felt purpose in giving back to other veterans through his music. Music is prescribed to patients as part of complementary care for help coping with symptoms of anxiety, mood, irritability, and insomnia, and my CD is given for musical meditation at home.

My song "Answering the Call" highlights the contributions of healthcare providers and employees answering the call to treat our nation's veterans. The song is included as part of the 75th Anniversary Celebration of the Veterans Health Administration.

Poetry is an additional tool that enhances the patient-centered experience in which patients feel listened to and their experience validated. Poignant accounts of trauma and grief kindled me to write poetry and share my work, which seemed to strengthen the doctor-patient relationship by forging an empathic connection. Patients find poetry to have therapeutic benefit; it serves as a springboard for future discussion, and they are also encouraged to write.

Healthcare professionals can harness the creative arts and talents they and their colleagues possess to explore unique ways to connect and partner with patients as a healing team, introducing a new dimension to the healthcare experience in a patient's journey to healing.

As chair of the American Medical Women's Association (AMWA) Music and Medicine Committee, physicians and medical students collaborate and are mentored to blend music in their personal and professional lives. They are "music ambassadors" in their own clinics and hospitals.

Composing AMWA's centennial theme song, "Physicians Healers," for the International Congress of AMWA and the Medical Women's International Association in New York was an honor. The song is a testament to the vision of trailblazing women leaders who paved the way for all women physicians to realize their dream of becoming doctors.

Witnessing the impact the pandemic has on healthcare workers and inspired by their dedication and selflessness, I wrote a song called "Healthcare Heroes."

"Physicians Healers and Healthcare Heroes" was developed as a YouTube video to pay musical and artistic tribute to the remarkable courage and compassion of healthcare providers during the COVID-19 pandemic and for their service every day. The YouTube video based on my songs features national and international women physicians, nurses, and healthcare providers. Women physicians sing with me on the track, as well as singers from Westminster Choir College. I composed a reflection on viola to conclude the video. "Physicians Healers and Healthcare Heroes" to commemorate the meaningful mission of physicians and healthcare heroes all over the globe through music. Together, they have risen to the challenge this crisis has presented— they have comforted the sick and dying, stayed at the bedside of those in need, and saved lives. As they guide and shine a light for others in the darkest of times, our healthcare heroes are beacons of light. We are eternally grateful for them.

My parents, grandparents, family, and an array of musical mentors taught me from a young age to pursue my dual passions and give to others through music, and that has been the greatest gift. Music lifts spirits; it is a conversation of souls, a connection of hearts, and a compelling expression of love and beauty.

My high school graduation page quoted romantic poet William Wordsworth, which speaks to the transcendent power of music, meant to be cherished and shared as a gift. "The music in my heart I bore, Long after it was heard no more."

Mary C. Rorro, D.O.
Psychiatry

LIFE CHOICES

"Jane died last night." His voice, though quiet, seemed strained.

"Are you all right?" I asked. There was a pause.

"She wouldn't let go. Do you remember when we were working out a few years ago, and you told me Jane looked as if she were going to fall over. She would have if the instructor hadn't told her to sit down. She was so angry with herself for not being able to go on. It was like that at the end. Her heart would stop for long periods, and then she would breathe, and it would start again. I finally had to tell her it was okay and that she should go to sleep."

Diagnosed with lymphoma four years ago, Jane had been at war with her disease since. She had lived longer than expected. She had been a fighter.

He wasn't telling me for my sake. I was listening because he needed to tell someone. She had not only been his wife; she had been his world. They had had one of those rare relationships where they had loved each other so deeply, it was often to the exclusion of the rest of the world. She had been awarded her black belt in karate the day before she died. She was fifty-two.

I had a few hours to kill before meeting my mentor at Swedish American Hospital, so I asked a physician I know to introduce me to someone in the ER whom I could follow. Whenever the books begin to get too heavy and the study hours too long, I head for the hospital to watch surgery or spend time in the ER following doctors. It helps me to remember that the practice of medicine involves taking care of people, not just their bodies.

For the first forty-five minutes, we had the normal whirlwind of fractures, hypoglycemic diabetics, patients in respiratory distress, and assorted minor difficulties. And then the call came over the radio. Fourteen-year-old male, gunshot wound to the head. He is posturing. ETA four minutes.

Four minutes of organized commotion later, I watched as a multitude of attendants swarmed over the body of a boy who had treated life as a game

92

and was losing. Quickly, nurses and technicians sliced his clothes away to gain access to life-sustaining blood vessels. I saw his body was profusely scarred by burns which had long since been treated and healed. The doctor called me to the head of the gurney and handed me a nasogastric tube. I told her I had never inserted one before, and she said that now was the time to learn. That's a bad sign. The only time a doctor wastes the time to show a medical student how to perform a procedure on a real patient in the ER is when that doctor knows there's no hope. It was then I noticed the large bump on the side of the boy's head where the bullet had lodged, pushing the skull outwards.

Outside, I overheard the paramedics talking about how the boy's seventeen-year-old brother had put the gun to his head and pulled the trigger in a game of Russian roulette. Later at Swedes, I heard the same paramedics telling a different audience. Though it made me a bit ill to hear it, I couldn't blame them; even the newspapers thought it a good sensationalistic story.

Driving home, I wondered how life can be viewed so differently by different people. How is it that one person fights tooth and nail to hold on to a frail, dying body, while someone else simply throws life away without a second thought? Why is it that often people don't fight to live until death comes calling?

A fourteen-year-old boy died last night. He hung on for three days but never awakened. Nothing was gained. Nothing was learned. No life was lived to its fullest. The struggle to live had come too late.

H.E. Guy Burman
University of Illinois College of Medicine at Rockford
Class of 1996

FULL CIRCLE

I was seven when my family moved from the bustling hub of Hudson, New York, to Ketchikan, Alaska—a rural island fishing town accessible only by ferry or float plane. The cross-country move was motivated largely by Dad's need to have a more balanced work and home life. The understaffed metropolitan hospital of Hudson left very little breathing room for being a father as well as a surgeon. On the day of my sister's adoption, Dad was supposed to have the whole day off. He ended up in the OR all morning and was able to meet us at the courtroom just in time to sign the adoption papers before heading back in for another case. By the time my sister was six months old, he had spent a total of ten waking hours with her. While he and my mother had anticipated the long hours and frequent 2 AM calls, this amount of unbalance between having a career and having a family was proving to be unmanageable. So, when the call came from PeaceHealth Ketchikan Medical Center to say that their current surgeon was about to retire, my family packed our bags and went.

My parents had met in Ketchikan almost fifteen years previously, when Dad took a year off from med school and Mom was working as a pediatric speech pathologist. They returned to the island years later to get married, but Dad's residency had pulled them back to Memphis and then New York, and they hadn't returned to the island since. Dad's decision to take a year off from medical school was prompted in part by the death of Jane, the close friend whose fight for life inspired his original submission to *Becoming Doctors*. I think her passing, in addition to all the other deaths he was witnessing as a medical student, brought to the surface questions about the nature of being a doctor that begged answering.

Dad is the third-generation product of a sort of father–son pipeline of physicians. His father was a pioneering heart surgeon and his father before

94

him had been the town doctor in Syracuse, New York. Dad had been on a straight path trajectory to becoming a physician himself since very early on, and I think the death of a close friend and the inability of modern medicine to prevent it prompted a bit of soul searching as to whether or not the path he was currently on was the right one to continue down. At the very least, I think he was feeling the need to go out and experience some life of his own before resigning himself to at least six more years of study. And so it was that my father, the twenty-five-year-old Ivy League grad, left medical school to gut sea cucumbers and camp out behind a gas station in rural southeast Alaska. Having spent a year living life and seeking answers among the black bears and commercial fishing boats, he went back to finish med school, start a family, and begin his career as a general surgeon. So, life went on, until the call came from PeaceHealth and my father returned to practice medicine in the very place he had gone many years ago to escape it.

For me, being the surgeon's daughter at a fifty-bed island clinic was an experience unique to any I had yet encountered in my young life. With few exceptions, I more or less had free rein of the place. My memories from PeaceHealth are of wandering through the ER with my pockets full of gumballs, blowing latex glove balloons and distributing them to nurses, peeping behind sterile-smelling curtains to chat with patients, and sitting out by the launchpad to watch the helicopter deliver patients from other islands. The convoluted multifacility complex of Columbia Memorial Hospital was replaced by a single building whose hallways I could navigate as well as any employee. Whereas the ER in Hudson had been marked by an ominous set of double doors from which Dad would briefly emerge in full scrubs to receive his brown bag lunch, in Ketchikan I could walk right in and deliver his lunches in person. Dad's starched shirts and ties were replaced by jeans and casual button downs, and he even grew a beard—something he would have considered very unprofessional back in New York. Instead of doing computer work in a large room shared by ten other people, Dad had his own little office with art on the walls (frequently mine or my sister's) and a desk drawer of goodies especially awaiting my visits. My interactions with Dad's work in Ketchikan were not limited to the hospital, either. He received frequent calls from friends or friends of friends in need and would often travel to their homes or the site of an injury to give assistance. He made routine trips to a smaller island nearby that had no resident surgeon, and my family would often come along with him on these journeys.

Our own kitchen table became the site of multiple minor procedures, as well. There would be a holler of "so-and-so is going to stop by to have his finger checked out!" and a few minutes later, there would be drop cloths and wound dressings scattered about the kitchen. I was frequently allowed onsite to hold gauze pads or fetch instruments, which made my eight-year-old self bubble with importance. I liked to be in the thick of it and was never easily deterred by the whole blood-and-guts aspect of the process. I was raised watching my neighbors gut fish and skin otters, after all.

Having such a close relationship with my father's work also gave me a unique perspective on what it meant to be the doctor of a rural community. There was a certain level of respect that came with being the only surgeon on the island that I haven't quite seen anywhere else he has worked. Whenever we went out, he would frequently be stopped by calls of "hey,f Doc!" followed by a friendly greeting and conversation. There was a sense of mutual respect and understanding that extended beyond the office and into daily life. In a world where you knew everyone and their neighbor, it was impossible not to have that deeper connection between patient and physician—the guy on your table one day could be the mechanic who fixed your outboard motor last week.

My father's practice in Ketchikan was one of community and of love. People gave what they had freely and with compassion, and he was certainly no exception. He encouraged people to give what they could and would frequently provide care for other than monetary compensation. Our home became filled with homemade jams, knitted hats, woven baskets, and carved bowls that patients had given in payment for their procedures. On one memorable occasion, Dad brought home three live five-foot-long king crabs a patient had proffered in exchange for his appendectomy.

Twenty-five years ago, my father wrote about death. While he has seen and dealt with much more of it in the years since writing that original piece, he's also experienced a fair amount of life. I wonder sometimes if it hadn't been for that year off from med school that eventually led to my family's move to Alaska, if Dad would have found the same sense of fulfillment with his career that he has now. While my family no longer lives in Ketchikan, he still carries on that unique sense of respect and community in his practice. Whether it's bringing homemade pho to his Vietnamese patient or making time to check in on recovering friends, I think the time spent at PeaceHealth enabled him in a way to go that extra mile that someone of a more traditional medical background might not consider.

Last summer, Dad was able to take a couple weeks off to go back up to Ketchikan and work as a locum. I got to travel with him—an echo of my years spent eagerly trailing at his heels through that same hospital as a child. The trip gave both of us the chance to reconnect with the island and gave me a new perspective on the influence a doctor can have on their community. As with any profession, I think as a doctor you eventually reach a point where you are compelled to look back and think "have I really done anything that has made a positive impact on the world?" In a community as small as Ketchikan, that impact is very tangible, and I hope that returning to it allowed my father to see the impact that he had made on it, and vice versa. I know I could.

Sarah Wendy Burman on behalf of H.E. Guy Burman, M.D.
General Surgery

A LONG-OVERDUE LETTER
TO AN OLD FRIEND

News from the abyss—or should it read as a note from a bottle— *lost on a forsaken island, send help!* Maybe the most appropriate beginning would be, *it seems like forever—I miss you much.*

> I gave my life to become the person I am right now. Was it worth it?
>
> —Richard Bach

So much has happened in the past months that I hardly know where to begin. In short, it has been amazing, treacherous, demeaning, stimulating, humiliating, painful, intriguing, humbling, beautiful, and horrible, and always incredibly intense. Sometimes overwhelmingly, the system is winning; it sucks the life out of us, changing us and challenging every belief we ever had, taking our humanness, and trampling it, stretching the limits of tolerance and stamina to render the lot of us sniveling fools. The most important lesson I have learned is that I must stay human in this system. Chance meetings or vacations have become telling experiences as I see old friends, people with the resources to love, and realize I have so fully lost touch with them, with you, that I cannot even share my experience so you can understand; so, I sit, smiling, uncomfortable, unable to reach out for rescue, thinking that to let my guard down in any realm would mean the demise of my career and my dreams. I know now I must try.

> Where is the Life we have lost living?
> Where is the wisdom we have lost in knowledge?
> Where is the knowledge we have lost in information?
>
> —T.S. Elliot

Your heart pounds as the mailman departs. The letter has arrived. It is a big envelope. You think maybe, could it be true, you, a doctor. Tearing nervously, anxiously, scanning the congenialities, you look for those key words, "Sorry, the committee . . ." or "Congratulations, the Medical College of . . . has accepted you for matriculation into. . . ." All respiration stops, and your heart, responding to the onslaught of hormones, flutters aimlessly; your brain throbs as it seeks to make sense of the ink images on the paper. In ironic ecstasy, a synapse between your neurons conveys the sought-after answer—you're in! Your life has changed immeasurably; you will never be the same.

> But how is the poor wretch to acquire the ideal qualifications that
> he needs in his profession?
> —Sigmund Freud, "Analysis Terminable and Interminable"

The first day of school, you enter the mysterious and enchanted world full of hope and intrigue, like the neonate who gasps for air as the placenta is cut—the rest of your life is excitingly ahead of you. And like that new child, you sense a terror, but you would rather fend it off with defenses of arrogance and fidelity so as to mask the enemy. Everything in the world seems in order, even romantic, as you acquire monumental textbooks full of the stuff of your dreams, as you muddle through the schedule exploring the new surroundings, as you awkwardly meet your fellow victims, and as you embark on the incredible journey of medicine. Later that day, you put the key they gave you into the large wooden door marked with a hazardous material sign to meet the first of many dead people who can hurt you more than you can imagine. You look on with bated breath as the quaint gentleman, who seems like a character you know very well out of some novel—only you can't decide if it's a Robert Fulghum novel or a Stephen King novel—pulls back the plastic to reveal a cadaver. There before you is a naked human, motionless, reeking of phenol and formalin, skin wrinkled and discolored, stiff and glazed. You make the mental mistake that this should not bother you for you are to be a doctor; and so, to distract yourself, you remember that so many people can only halfheartedly dream of being in medical school, but you are here, and in that you find solace. You lose such a tiny fragment of yourself in that moment, it is wholly imperceivable, like the silent genetic mutation that causes a single cancerous cell to grow years later uncontrolled, slowly and painfully gnawing the life out of that individual.

Convinced of the honor of the profession, enraptured by the mystique that medicine evokes, and proud of your vocation, you set out to learn all you can. Like a dry sponge in an ocean, you swell courageously with information that seems always relevant and fascinating until every pore of your being is engorged and a wave crashes your tiny remains into the drowning darkness. Oh, sure, there is a lot of information that you need to be proficient at your job; well suck it up, others have done it. Yes, but all have scars. With each fact, the horror of mistake looms over your head— if I forget just one enzyme, if I misidentify that nerve, if I use too much of that drug, if I was sleepy the day that your disease was taught, and if my mind can't hold the volumes of new terms and concepts daily hurled on these, the innocent, I can hurt you, I can kill you, my patient; you, the one I so honestly want to serve; you, for whom I cried that *if I can ease one life the aching, or cool one pain, or help one fainting robin unto his nest again, I shall not live in vain* (Emily Dickinson); you, for whom I so naively care. Soon, though, the patient and his problems will become part of the system; she will lose her humanity, just as surely as I will lose mine; he, she, "it" will become part of my nightmare.

aegrescit medendo—the treatment may be worse than the disease

There on the table lies Mr. RJ (to protect the innocent, we can't even use names; or is it to protect our fragile egos?). Rather we call him the gomer in room six, the S/P CABG c 2° DVT/PE and CVA (that is, status postcoronary artery bypass graft with secondary deep vein thrombosis, causing a pulmonary embolism and concomitant cerebral vascular accident)—translated, a body without a brain, a heart that we prodded and cut and supposedly repaired, and a remnant of an organism kept alive entirely by our technology whom we refer to by his disease, most of which was never his condition until we, in our wisdom and cruel altruism, took to beneficently bestow it upon him. And because we were too busy "caring" for our patient, we never spoke about "do not resuscitate orders" to his son, who fondly thinks him the kindest soul and best fisherman in all of Round Valley; to his wife, who lovingly shared the last forty-three years, or to the rest of his tearful family, who were isolated from this dying man by punctuated visiting hours in the intensive care unit so we could do our most virtuous job. I now pound on the chest of this vestige of organic material, thinking my actions certainly nonmaleficent. We work the code; that is, perform actions for which charges of rape and assault would be filed outside of the hallowed halls of the hospital, in a protocol to restart his failing heart and breathe oxygen into his shriveling lungs. Finally, disappointed, we "call it"—let the poor soul finish this stage of his journey; we are despondent, for we have failed to ensure immortality. Is it any wonder I am no longer what I once was?

> The patient is the one with the disease.
> —Samuel Shem, rule IV, *The House of God*

Or am I the one with the disease? Without exception, each of us would benefit from ardent psychiatric intervention. Yet, I am thankful for the journey. Amazing as it seems, in any state of stress and pain can come profound insight and growth. I was entirely unprepared for what I was about to partake of. My selfishness, my barriers to love, and my weaknesses were all nicely masked in the ease with which I had stumbled along up to now in the world. I have had to redefine purpose and meaning in my life; I have learned to expect very little and celebrate all that is beautiful. Our friendship was indeed that—and I am sorry for not including you up to now. *Love* You!

~~medical student~~ recovering human being

Richard A. Mularski
University of Arizona College of Medicine
Class of 1996

TWENTY-FIVE YEARS LATER
ANOTHER HEARTFELT AND BIT REFLECTIVE
LETTER TO MY GOOD FRIEND

Dear friend:

It's been good being in touch over the years and sharing the richness of life, love, loss, and the beauty of simply being . . . that is being alive in moment-to-moment awareness of our humanness. Like I often relate at the culmination of end-of-life experiences with patients and their families, it has been a privilege and pleasure to walk along the journey with you.

One day you finally knew what you had to do, and began,
though the voices around you kept shouting their bad advice-
though the whole house began to tremble, and you felt the old tug
at your ankles.
'Mend my life!' each voice cried.
But you didn't stop. You knew what you had to do,
though the wind pried with its stiff fingers at the very foundations,
though their melancholy was terrible.
It was already late enough, and a wild night,
and the road full of fallen branches and stones.
But little by little, as you left their voices behind,
the stars began to burn through the sheets of clouds,
and there was a new voice which you slowly recognized as your own,
that kept you company as you strode deeper and deeper into the world,
determined to do the only thing you could do-
determined to save the only life you could save.

— *The Journey* by Mary Oliver

Medical school is an amazing, humbling, and incredibly intense step, but really just the start of a journey—the isolation and insecurity as a student that led to our distance a quarter century ago created opportunity to open to grow and embrace all of the vocation of being a physician. As a health sciences pupil, one may emotionally feel the enormity of the task to become a care provider and might just be paying attention enough to embrace the responsibility of the sacred mission to walk with others as healer and doctor.

> We work in the dark—we do what we can—we give what we have.
> Our doubt is our passion, and our passion is our task. The rest is the madness of art.
>
> —Henry James

The practice of medicine—appreciate that we call it "practice," as our work must always be approached with humility and as the search for an ongoing expansion of our knowledge and experience—has afforded me much more than I could have expected. Happy to say I would do it all again . . . and hope for the same mistakes, achievements, joys, sorrows, wild course deviations, and titillating opportunities that, just as in training sometimes felt like trying to drink from a fire hose, has always left me satiated. Recall how we discussed selfishness, barriers, and weaknesses . . . that felt so limiting as a student—indeed these were the attitudes and sensibilities that made it possible to espouse intentionality and the real experience of our lives.

> When I see I am nothing, that is wisdom.
> When I see I am everything, that is love.
> And between these two, my life flows.
>
> —Sri Nisargadatta Maharaj

Wonderful mentors planted small seeds along the way like Tom's admonition (residency director, paraphrased), "You will and should continue to feel there is always too much to know, but if you approach each patient with the dedication and compassion you would for a loved one, like your own mom, you'll both take great care of those you are gifted to serve and learn what you need to know." Others opened doors, encouraged me to say yes a lot, and follow through, to think about systems, and to always look for improvement in the quality of care and the patient experience. Am I the same person I was back then? I'd have to say yes and more for the chances to grow and evolve into the person I am now. If I could have the foresight of current wisdom to send a message to the younger me, I'd probably just do as I try with every trainee—send encouragement and be grateful for the passion and engagement in all of it.

> Helping, fixing, and serving represent three different ways of seeing life. When you help, you see life as weak. When you fix, you see life as broken. When you serve, you see life as whole. Fixing and helping may be the work of the ego, and service the work of the soul.
> —Rachel Naomi Remen

You might remember that American Medical Student Association T-shirt I wore until threadbare that was embroidered with "To cure sometimes, to heal often, to care always." Simple ardors like that have helped make the voyage honest; keeping them as daily reminders facilitates keeping it real and refreshing. Having friends like you to share nonmedical stories and ask the silly questions you still do of my work, colleagues who were happy to go have coffee or play scrabble after a twelve-hour shift and debrief about giving news of that horrible diagnosis to that young man yesterday and how the family (and I and our staff) really took that older women's death hard, a loving wife who passionately shares our hospital work and sometimes even the same patients, and a practice of mindfulness and athletics are all part of the modus operandi that continues to sustain, heal, and motivate me. The experiences have led to a work life principally grounded in being a compassionate practitioner of medicine, enhanced by laboring as a scientist and quality improvement steward, and rooted in trying to be a good human.

> Our deepest fear is not that we are inadequate. Our deepest fear is that we are powerful beyond measure. It is our light, not our darkness, that most frightens us. We ask ourselves: Who am I to be brilliant, gorgeous, talented, and fabulous? Actually, who are you not to be? You are a child of God. Your playing small doesn't serve the world. There is nothing enlightened about shrinking so that other people won't feel insecure around you. We are born to manifest the glory of God that is within us. It is not just in some of us; it's in

everyone. And as we let our own light shine, we unconsciously give other people permission to do the same. As we are liberated from our own fear our presence automatically liberates others.

—Marianne Williamson in *A Return to Love* as quoted by Nelson Mandela in his inaugural speech, 1994

So lovely to share again, and looking forward to visiting soon. We can toast the new achievement of your daughter, reflect on the passing of our old friend, share stories of our newest aching body part, and smile together for all we've known and done. So, when your other kid asked me about going to med school, I simply said—don't do it lightly, but be light as you do it—bring compassion to all, including yourself—be collegial—celebrate life—have an amazing journey.

Love, me

Richard A. Mularski, M.D.
Pulmonary & Critical Care Medicine

VIEW FROM ELSEWHERE

I can see you in your gray-blue scrubs and oversized goggles. You look slightly panicked, the way I used to when I had four hundred runs to make and it was sleeting outside. I once lived in that body, lying there, skewered with scalpels and unprofessionally skinned. I wanted to tell you that it's all right that you're doing what you're doing. I gave myself to you. I shouldn't say self; I gave you this contraption with one bad lung, an oblong hernia, and acceptable muscles. This contraption that was once perfect, and like a Rube Goldberg machine, was made up of odd and uncomplimentary parts.

Look at my heart up-close so you can see the route the blood ran, the foramen ovale of my stork beak youth, and the bicuspid parachute that secured no return to sender. I still don't know how it continued for so long to ribbon up its package from the lungs and parcel it all over the body, even to the most remote, the most tiny, and the most hidden-away cell. How, minute by minute, by pen pals of electrical charge, it sent oxygen visiting every home in this town.

If my heart could be the best postman in Govans for seventy-two years, think what the soul of my heart could do. How far it could reach. Its redness and possibility. And those love letters still pass hands, though my heart doesn't beat anymore, though you hold it, rinse its ventricles, and note the circuit the sinus turns.

It's all right, too, that you take out my brain, that you cup it in your hands like bread left out in the rain. It has more folds in it than any mortal baker could ever braid. More pages in its folds than are pressed into a thousand Sears Roebuck catalogues. These logs, though, don't claim pleasure or bargains or even a sale. They are words and they are my stories, and though they, in a way, lie buried in the tissue you're holding, there, in order to see the nerves and the sulci and the circle of Willis, they're also carved out, drawn up, and written in the minutes of the world.

It's all right, too, that you weep a little, going home, smelling like form-aldehyde, tired from lectures and saddened by what you've sawed and cut and scraped. Saddened by what you've seen and felt. It's all right that you think of me. Who I was. Who lost me. Who delivered and who loved me. Who sits around a table, warm under the old brass lamp, and remembers something I said once, that old brick-walk jig, the bubblegum smell of my clothes. Who misses my mornings, my dreams, and my scattered smile.

Melissa Marks Sparrow
Johns Hopkins University School of Medicine
Class of 1998

I Have Intubated Children

I had been grappling with how I had changed as an emergency department physician in the past few years, and the providential nature of her outreach corralled my scattered outward searching into personal contemplation. I reread my submission to *Becoming Doctors* from twenty-five years ago, a fictional piece about a student's first exposure to death in anatomy class, and the young writer reached forward to me through time. Her words comforted me as they expressed sorrow for the death of a stranger and gratitude for the gift of his body. She reminded me that writing could help me to understand, to grieve, and to love. Rereading "View from Elsewhere" encouraged me to pick up words again.

I will begin with the blue star creeper. If I keep my eyes fixed on the staccato of spring blue, I can stand, for a moment, and breathe. My colleague allowed me the gift of respite—a respite I did not know my body would insist upon and has never insisted upon before. I have been doing this medical work a long time—almost twenty years—and done so within the walls of a pediatric emergency department that has become like another home to me: walls decorated by art collected from a local elementary school when we were a brand-new pediatric ED, my own children's art among them. Also, my father's art, his abstract *retablos* that children can reach out to and touch as they walk along the corridor.

My eyes wander to the trophy of the daffodil and its ruffled plate—daffodils in bunches planted in the way I could never quite accomplish in my own garden, perfectly apportioned. My heart beats in my throat. I am sweating. I have done this many, many times before. I have intubated children, choreographed toddlers into positions to protect their airways—passages of life—from the slippage of bottle caps, compressed chests to inner drum rhythms, *stayin' alive, stayin' alive,* and muscled my mouth over the mouth and nose of a cyanotic infant clasped in her mother's arms. I have stood at the frontier between life and death and performed in ways that have been called heroic by some, although, to me, *heroic* is a misplaced word for one's daily work, that for which I have been trained. I acknowledge, however, that my ability to care for acutely ill children and to lead, think, act, and *save* has crystallized, over the years, in solutions of risk and fear.

This time, my patient was a boy, a young man really, who presented with a terrible headache and what appeared to be a momentary seizure, a flutter of the eyes. This time, it could have been any boy, any toddler, a school-age child, a near man, as he was—the point being, he was young, my patient, and at risk. A CT scan revealed a cerebral sinus venous thrombosis—another passage of life potentially obstructed, another something standing between this and that, whom the patient was then and whom he might become, the world his family lived in and the rules they abided by then, and the ones that might reshape their world. I stood between this and that, between now and then; I and two nurses, a tech, medical systems, and physicians with the capacity to intervene surgically in a way that I could not, all those elements of medical care that I fully acknowledge, but so too I acknowledge my exquisite responsibility to orchestrate that moment. At this hour, on this day, I was the orchestra leader, the conductor, the concertmaster. I held the baton for this boy's brain and, therefore, his life.

I ordered antiepileptics for J to assure no seizures in transport, all sirens blaring. While waiting for the Keppra to be tubed from pharmacy, his eye strayed in a way that flagged for Ativan. Gina, the nurse, pushed the medication. J's eyes closed, but he continued to breathe gently and fully. Roxanne, another nurse, attended to his IV lines. Time stood on a cliff edge, an edge that I am normally quite comfortable with, as I walk with time, the widest berth of my foot aligned with its farthest boundary, not looking left, not looking right, only straight ahead.

His parents. I could give a million descriptions, I could tell you this and I could tell you that, but what has always stood out to me is my level of knowing and parents' level of knowing and the chasm in between. Panic, trust, distrust, desperation, confidence, anger, numbness, shock, or any combination thereof fill the space of that chasm like a volatile gas. My job is to remain still, to breathe amidst the gas, slow everything down, my respiratory rate, my heartbeat, my thoughts, my words, my actions. Slow. Everything. Down. While functioning at top speed. Inform, but do not overinform, emanate compassion, but avoid the realm of emotion that might weaken my capacity to think.

I speak directly to J, my voice upbeat, clear, familiar with being a mom of a boy this age, familiar with concealing my own personal terror while holding others clear of it. "Do you have any questions right now about what is happening?" I ask. He shakes his head. "I'm good." His face appears calm; wringing hands belie his assertion.

Once transport courses down the hall and out, I turn to walk away from the central nurses' station. My head is light and blood pools in all the wrong places. Now, my head is not light, but flattened by air with the density of cement. Blood is leaking out of me. Nausea tornadoes my stomach. Another doctor has arrived, and I ask her if I can step away.

"You look pale," she says.

In this hospital park called Blue Bell Park, even though the ground-cover flowers are not blue bells but blue star creepers, I can't shake the nausea, can't yank myself out of that place I descended into as I took care of J, a place I can no longer go safely, I am coming to understand. I don't want to return to the emergency department. I want to stay by the small wooden bridge and the trees casting shadows on the paths woven among the shade plants. There, that place, is proximal to death, or the possibility of death, and so is near my son, my son's death, which I have not even begun to comprehend. How can I function in a space that is suddenly so deep and vast and dark? How can I ask for trust in me, in my capacity to run a code, to take a collision of circumstances and hold them steady when I have none in myself?

I walk back to the pediatric unit, swiping my card with the picture of my technologically widened face, and slip into the bathroom to wipe a makeup wand under each eye. You would think I would wear waterproof mascara. But I don't. I apply lipstick. I am known for that, disappearing and resurfacing, ready to tackle a stormy situation with an unhappy parent, with fresh lipstick applied. I return to the doctors' work cubby—we call it that because it is honestly that small—and sit down to complete the chart. My cubbymate is of the gentlest nature. She gives me space and understanding. I tuck my purse under the desk.

Everyone here gives me space. The nurses, the techs, the doctors. I feel their support around me like invisible stakes in a garden. They know I cannot speak of my son and do not ask me to. It is all so fresh. Although when I do say something small, briefly reveal the grief with which I am living, they look up tenderly and listen. They know, I am sure, that certain situations trigger outstanding pain.

I don't know if I can do this job anymore.

My son had been mentally ill for six years, with gradually worsening paranoia that was eventually diagnosed as schizophrenia, when he ended his own life by suicide. His world was closing in on him, his hopes for a normal life were extinguished, his capacity for relationships except for immediate family members destroyed by the disease consuming his brain. His capacity for relationships with those who most loved him were also becoming compromised, as the paranoia was entering into his perception of even his immediate family. He was suffering from headaches that made him feel like he was having "brain bleeds." The medications he had been forced to take for years, with his own mother administering injections at times, made him feel inhuman. And so he made the decision only he could make, and which I fully understand, even though it broke my heart.

My son wanted his body given to science. Though no organs could be saved, we donated his body to scientific research through the Anatomy Gifts Registry, a nonprofit Maryland-based organization that facilitates whole body donation for purposes of furthering medical science and research. He wanted no funeral, no memorial, just to disappear "the way David Bowie did," he wrote in his "Five Wishes," an advanced directive I had actually asked all of us (Dad and sister too) to fill out because of my work with palliative care in the hospital. Fill in, fill out, what odd words to describe the expression of one's death wishes. Of course, I never imagined I would be referring to his directives. I did not recognize, as he asked question after question and insisted on no life support measures given certain conditions, his plan.

My son clearly wanted to minimize the pain his death would cause, if such an idea can even be considered by a parent, by going to a nearby state, assuring no one else could be hurt by his action, and that he would be immediately identified by whoever found him or saw him. I believe now, in retrospect, that he needed us as a family to love him enough to allow him this exit. The end of his suffering. The cessation of further loss.

We did not abide by "no memorial" though. We needed a ritual to remember him; our family and our community needed to remember who my son was when he was well, celebrate that person who was so painfully taken from himself and from us.

I picked up my son's ashes myself with a friend who is a fellow pediatrician and a pastor. They weighed almost as much as he did when he was born. I held the square wooden box on my lap the way I might have held a small infant, a treasure, something with which I was irrevocably connected. My friend made small talk. She, a doctor, colleague, and the mother of three boys, was a brave and uncompromising friend, one among the majority of my friends—not all—who could manage her discomfort in order to be with me. The impact, at the time, of what was happening, I could not process.

What I do know, at this moment, is that I have changed. The juxtaposition of what has happened in my life, the illness my son lived and died with, an illness that afflicted our family and tore it apart, and my professional identity as someone who saves lives, as someone who believes in the power of western medicine to help and even rectify, do not align in the way they used to. Unrest weighs on me like too much knowledge. How do I take what I know, what is integral to who I am as a doctor and mother, intertwined identities, and shape them into something that honors my son? That continues his story and allows me to speak the truth of mine?

Move, Melissa, move, something tells me. Memories linger like burns in this emergency department that was once like another home: my children visiting to pick up keys or credit cards. MaryLouise is locked out. Russell needs the car. Phone calls imploring me to sign out and come home. Dad is cooking venison again. MaryLouise needs to make madeleines for French class tomorrow; who has a madeleine pan? Russell chipped a tooth. The dog ate his boutonniere. I miss you Mommy and am making up reasons why. Mommy, please come home. When are you coming home?

And then there were the later calls, as illness snaked its way through our home, Ned disappearing, unable to strategize; Russell withdrawing into fears of attack and disease; my daughter simply trying to survive.

One night, when I first started working at this hospital and a distinct pediatric emergency department had not yet opened, and we pediatricians worked as pure hospitalists, my son and daughter spent the night with me in my tiny call room. A hurricane whirled outside, yet we were safe, perhaps the safest I have ever felt, curled up with my two children in a profoundly uncomfortable bed—barely able to sleep so squeezed was I between their sprawling forms. Not many calls to the floor or the ED that hurricane night. In the morning, outside the call room window, you could see Blue Bell Park, some branches down, not much else visible but sheets of rain.

Melissa Marks Sparrow, M.D.
Pediatrics

MRS. S.

I keep thinking
of the woman they wheeled in today
Her nightgown up high around her legs, one eye patched, the other blind
She didn't realize we addressed her
ten students
sitting against the wall and on the heater
We still questioned, she answered any answer
and yawned and said she's accepted it all
Her husband's death, her son's murder, her own fatal illness
and asked to be wheeled away.

Rachel Burdick Vinkey
State University of New York Health Science Center at Brooklyn
College of Medicine
Class of 1997

TWENTY-FIVE YEARS

When the faces in my drawings from more than twenty-five years ago look back at me now, I see a wariness in their eyes, a sense of alienation, frustration, even anger. My poem from the same period, "Mrs. S.," resonates flatness, resignation, and disconnection.

My journey as an artist has paralleled my journey as a healer. In high school, college, and early medical school, my artwork was sharp, intense, realistic, or surreal, often with darker themes. In college, as my study of Western philosophy gave way to the study of poetry and Eastern philosophy, my tight, hyper-realistic artwork loosened. Along the way, abstract painting, collage, and photography became my preferred modes of self-expression. A stiff and dualistic worldview gave way to a more holistic one.

After the grind of medical school and the exhaustion of internship, psychiatry residency felt like a breath of fresh air. Communication and connection were emphasized, and I was encouraged to develop my intuition. The study of the brain fascinated me. I was excited to look at the human experience from all the angles: biological, psychological, and social, and always through the lens of intimate connection. Sitting with each patient in therapy felt like standing before a completely unique painting, sensing all elements and layers, a wholeness inclusive of complexity.

Throughout my training, I took every opportunity for research or in practicum to study creativity and healing. This included an art group on an inpatient psychiatry prison ward, where patients filled up a wall with their drawings and paintings; individual art therapy with a seven-year-old boy who used construction paper to construct what he needed from the world; and an outpatient art group where I sat side by side with young

115

adult patients, making collage and crafts, later inviting them to fill out questionnaires about their experiences. My work also included research papers on meaning and maturation in children's art, psychopharmacology, and creativity, and a research review of the biopsychosocial impact of creativity on healing.

After residency, a move across the country, a few years in academic medicine, and the birth of my daughter, I chose a career in private practice. I love having the autonomy to meet each patient where they are and to take the time I need to get to know them. I enjoy seeing their issues through multiple lenses: assessing physical health, possible psychopharmacological interventions, family of origin issues and current relationships, along with their strengths and desires for the future. I see everyone for therapy as well as medication management and do not do short medication checks. This allows me to practice in the holistic manner I prefer.

My own wellness practices now greatly influence my work with patients. As a former high school and college runner, I still run daily after more than forty years. I am very aware of exercise's mental and physical benefits and try to encourage my patients to find ways to move their bodies joyfully. I am very grateful for the wise input of a gifted chiropractor, acupuncturist, and body worker who have shared knowledge that I could not have found in traditional Western medicine. Yoga, meditation, and qigong are now regular practices for me. When appropriate, I suggest these to my patients. Whether I do so directly or not, practices of embodiment suffuse my work. I encourage body mindfulness: getting patients to feel their bodies, to sense into them, and to breathe and tap into their body's intuition. I have found that this sort of deep body awareness is a shortcut to mental and physical health. Research has borne out the powerful effects of such practices. Centers that study complementary medicine have begun to crop up at medical schools across the country. The powerful impact of meditation, qigong, and yoga have all been well-documented.

In recent years, I have also come to see the profound healing impact of nature: a simple walk in the woods or a few minutes of gazing up into the night sky can elicit feelings of calm and wholeness, a sense of one's place as a part of something greater. Time in an urban forest near my home is important to me. Recent research has also pointed to the health benefits of time in the natural world and spiritual practice. I strongly encourage my patients to integrate nature into their lives however they can and to find a way to honor whatever spiritual impulse they might have.

My lifelong exploration of healing has led me to some old-fashioned, even ancient practices. I believe that these ancient practices, paradoxically, are the future.

Rachel B. Vinkey, M.D.
Psychiatry

END OF THE HONEYMOON

The events of the past week have ended the honeymoon of my first year in medical school. During the first two weeks, I was actually having fun with the problem-based learning cases, so much so that I felt guilty, since fun and medical school are not normally uttered in the same sentence. Even though patients in our cases have died, it was only on paper. During the past week though, I've had the cold reality of medicine rammed down my throat. My girlfriend's father has been in a hospital for two-and-a-half months waiting for a donor heart. Monday, the news came through that he was finally going to undergo transplant surgery. This was a long-awaited relief—the end was in sight and he would soon be home.

By Wednesday, the transplanted heart was rejected, quite possibly because of poor judgment on the part of a physician. It turns out that normally, transplant patients are kept on a respirator for twenty-four to thirty-six hours. His respirator was removed after twenty hours, at two o'clock in the morning, no less, without the approval of the attending physician. The transplanted heart failed within two hours. An emergency biventricular assist device was implanted, but by this time, other organs had been irreparably compromised. It later came to light that the donor heart had an abnormal EKG from the start. By Thursday, he was in a coma and by Friday, he was declared brain dead. Life support was removed. This is a harsh reality of medicine, one which I had mistakenly thought I was prepared for.

In what seemed a surreal, almost voyeuristic manner, I was forced to experience firsthand many of the nonscientific aspects of medicine that we are taught up front in the problem-based learning curriculum. I saw how physicians break bad news to the affected family, how physicians can at times keep the family in the dark and even appear to change their story as the gravity of the situation becomes apparent, how social workers intervene and interact with the families, and how consent forms are used, even at two o'clock in the morning. Most importantly, I saw how a family is affected by an operation gone wrong and how any patient can be one of the unlucky ones who falls into the unfortunate 5 percent of an operation with a 95 percent success rate.

These events do not change my conviction that I want to become a physician, although I am left with some residual doubt as to how well I will cope with the imperfection of current medical practice. I cannot help but feel a cumulative disgust with the failings of medicine, although I'm not sure toward what or whom my disgust is directed. This is manifested by my lack of desire to dive into our newest paper case.

Many times, a physician's best efforts are not enough to stop the steady progression of a disease. I'm sure that virtually all physicians must deal with the death of a patient at some time in their careers. To be directly responsible must be devastating.

Often, in our modern incarnation of medical practice, what could be termed "medical heroics" are performed in a last-chance effort to fight a particularly critical disease process. I think we must not lose sight of the patient's best interests in such situations. No patient should unwittingly be turned into a guinea pig for trying out new techniques or pushing outward the envelope of acceptable criteria. Sometimes, a physician should let nature take its course and accept that we do not have an unlimited supply of miracles.

From this ordeal, several general messages emerged for me. It's better to err on the side of caution—if the patient were your father or mother, how would you proceed? Be honest with the family and keep them posted if you said you would—all respect for a physician is lost when the physician backpedals or appears to lie. Finally, when things go wrong, someone is going to be devastated—this is a fact of medicine, one which a good physician must always be aware of but must not be afraid of.

Keith Scott Dickerson
Medical College of Pennsylvania
Class of 1997

SILVER ANNIVERSARY—
END OF THE
HONEYMOON REVISITED

There is a profound naivety and act of faith when going into medicine. We cannot reasonably conceive what it will be like to have the immense responsibility that a clinician has, to actually be all that goes into being The Doctor. Practicing medicine is a true spiritual journey, forging each of our spirits in an ongoing crucible of grave decisions, uncertainties, paradoxes, and polarities. Choosing to study family medicine, we have a theoretic, non-lived notion that continuity of care and taking care of multiple family members will be a wonderful thing. The paradox is as medical students, we usually have, at most, a couple of months of patient continuity. Even during residency, you just barely get a taste of it, at most for a three-year stretch, often for not much more than a year. Those one- to three-year experiences can be quite meaningful, but not until after residency do you truly have the opportunity to experience continuity of care over many years.

One of my big focuses has been quality and patient safety, especially critical thinking and system optimization. I now realize that passion took hold early in medical school with several medical misadventure experiences in my personal life, one of which I wrote about in *End of the Honeymoon*. Myriad patient cases have now informed my practice of medicine, helping me gain perspective along my path of self-actualization. The virtues that lead toward excellence in care have become more apparent, while the edges of harsh judgment have been softened. An enduring career in medicine is like a marriage, and many of the same virtues that lead to success apply. If untoward events were the end of the honeymoon for me twenty-five years ago, many intervening events have led to a long-lasting and rewarding relationship with medicine, in particular the acceptance of and, at times, embracing of death. I offer these vignettes in virtue.

Humility—I thought you were old and not long for this world when I met you fifteen years ago during an admission under my care for RVR atrial fibrillation. Over the subsequent years, you amazed and inspired me with your resilience and spunk, relative health, and continued social engagement well into your nineties. It was truly my pleasure to be there for you after the tragic accidental injury that led you to conclude you had had enough—life was complete and you did not have the will to recuperate. I attended to you until the very end when you, being of sound mind and tranquil equanimity, decided you wanted to be admitted to inpatient hospice. At the bedside on the last day, I asked if you had any final thoughts for me or your loving family who were at your bedside. You succinctly smiled and kindly stated, "I love you all and it's going to be all right."

Conscientiousness, compassion, and vulnerability—I cared for multiple members of your extended family, all who have since passed while under my care, and now it is just you and me every three months, with occasional reminiscence of those who have gone before. You don't know this, but I often share with residents the story of your cousin's death while under my care—it's the least I can do. Their mother, your aunt, trusted me with their care. They became ill, and I didn't recognize soon enough the out-of-control spiral the cardiac medications had entered with the kidneys. I share the story yearly to atone and to hopefully help another clinician avoid the vicious cycle I misjudged.

You are reasonably healthy with just a couple well-managed chronic diseases, but I make it a common practice to have candid end-of-life discussions with my willing older patients. We had this discussion several years ago, which is documented in your chart, with a specific example that I use to bring home the reality of how DNR/DNI and my recent favorite, AND—Allow a Natural Death—actually play out. You have this exact event happen and I know your wishes, which I can confidently discuss with your MDPOA who has been so unexpectedly called to duty. We honor your wishes for no life-sustaining treatments in the face of unrecoverable neurologic damage. A family chapter rich with continuity is closed.

Being Present—A pleasant and polite early baby boomer, you always called me "Doctor" in a formal, respectful tone. After I would ask a question, you would begin with "Doctor . . . ," "Doctor, thank you for . . . ,"

"Doctor, I want you to know . . ." Yet there was an undeniable warmth as we talked about your outdoor adventures, and your eyes lit up when you spoke about your family.

The combination of myelodysplastic cancer resulting in chronic anemia would prove too taxing for your chronic heart failure. We are all relatively poor at prognosticating, yet my sense was that you had less time than the six to eight months your latest oncologist had recently quoted and certainly much less than the couple years that a recent hospice consultation had suggested. You came close to dying shortly after midnight one night while I happened to be on call at the hospital for our teaching service. After the resident contacted me, I initially considered going back to sleep, but then I roused myself, went to your bedside, and we had an intensely meaningful twenty-minute moment, coaxing your heart back from the brink, barely able to keep your blood pressure over 90/60, yet needing the cardiac medications. I was moments from calling your spouse in the wee hours of the morning when your chest pain completely abated after a series of medications at about 1 AM. We sat in the dim silence for a while—you had proven just how tenuous your situation was.

Over the last few days, your family had been able to arrive and say goodbye. There was no unfinished business, financial or familywise. I had asked the mortal questions Atul Gawande recently compiled. Your answers surprised me. What would a good day look like? Driving with your spouse into the desert, finding a nice spot, making a fire out of cedar, and roasting a chicken. In the end, you were unable to do this. You died within a day of being discharged to go home, but having the conversation and exploring what was important to you was the important part. For me, this is why I went into medicine—to allow myself to experience moments like this and being there for a patient and their family, even in the middle of the night. Over a remarkable two-day inpatient stretch, you and your spouse would go from nonacceptance that the end was near to complete acceptance, turning off the implanted defibrillator in your chest, and going home with hospice services.

Nurturing Relationship—When I inherited you as a patient fifteen years ago, you were on several hundred PO MSO4 equivalents per day, yet working full time. We sparred for years over the benefits and practicalities of tapering your doses versus your reality of ongoing, existential chronic pain. Through your numerous, almost cat-of-nine-lives dire medical events, we reached an uneasy peace and tapered most of your medication to more reasonable dosages. I balanced your genuine acts of kindness with a nagging sense of, perhaps, being manipulated for my continued much lower dose prescriptions. When the final devastating illness struck and rapidly progressed, you asked me if I would speak for perhaps five minutes at your memorial service. Boundaries and Oslerian objective detachment be damned—how could I say no? Is this not what we go into medicine for—to have meaningful relationships, meaningful enough to give a memorial? I was introduced as "The Doctor" and spoke my piece mostly reading passages from your own words that you had shared with me in your handwritten cursive letters and notes.

My dual career as a clinician and graduate medicine educator has evolved in such an unanticipated, wonderful way. Either career would be sufficiently rewarding, but having both in synergy and synchronicity is a true blessing. I now recognize that many of the case examples I use in my teaching with the residents are a form of atonement for less-than-optimal care and medical misadventures that I have witnessed and, yes, clinical misjudgments I have been part of. We owe it to our patients to not just learn from their predicaments but to try incrementally and respectfully to improve the care for the next patient. A rewarding career in clinical medicine needs to be nurtured like a marriage. Reflecting back on a twenty-five-year career affirms that choosing a career in medicine has given me more purpose that I could have imagined, humbled me in the best way, and accomplished what I hoped the career would—unending opportunities for learning and growth as I walk my spiritual journey.

Keith Scott Dickerson, M.D.
Family Medicine

Trapped on the First-Year Roller Coaster

Late last night, R asked me, "So, why did you *really* decide to go to medical school?" The question didn't surprise me too much. About once a week, I find myself lying in the temporary security of R's arms, complaining about my lack of commitment as a medical student. Without thinking too much, I answered, "Because I needed some direction in my life." I am currently a twenty-one-year-old, rebellious medical school student with plenty of direction but little conviction.

Why does anyone decide to go to medical school? It certainly isn't for those "oh-so-stimulating" biochemistry lectures that drag on for hours, or those long afternoons spent digging through layers of greasy fascia in gross lab. From talking to my classmates about this question and reflecting on my own history, I've concluded that many medical students had traumatic childhood experiences which transformed them into the driven people that they are today. For example, I was a social outcast from kindergarten to about eighth grade. I used to dread getting up and going to school each morning because I knew that vicious little kids were waiting there to torment me. Instead of relying on friends, who were few and far between, to bolster my self-esteem, I turned to my schoolwork. In early childhood, I threw myself headfirst into books and isolation. My manic dedication to academic achievement propelled me through Yale University (in three years) and into medical school. Everything happened so quickly that I never had time to think about what I was doing. I remember that in my senior year of college, I felt that I was caught in the middle of a gigantic snowball, rolling faster and faster down an avalanche. Now that the application whirlwind is over, I'm finally opening my eyes to my situation and questioning the values that got me this far. No longer does academic achievement seem that important. Rather, developing strong relationships with my peers and living for the moment are my primary concerns. Needless to say, these goals don't make me a particularly good student. At this very moment, I'm skipping a physiology class to write. Ah well.

I'm not the only one in my class whose childhood played a strong role in facilitating the route to medical school. In fact, most of my classmates have been through their own harrowing experiences. In the late hours of the evening, my friend/lover R shocked me with his story. When he was about three years old, R's parents decided to get divorced. Unfortunately, the divorce dragged on for over ten years. Once, during the custody battle, R was even pulled into the courtroom to select his preferred parent. Luckily, the judge refused to subject such a young child to the ordeal of testifying. Considering his stormy youth, R has done remarkably well. Following his college career, where he rowed crew to his heart's content, he received an MA in history. He's looking forward to the day when he can finally integrate medicine with history, his first love.

Another friend, G, comes from an entirely different, if not equally challenging, background. When I think about G's experience, I am amazed that she is here at all. Most medical students receive a great deal of support from their parents, unlike G. The eldest of ten children, G comes from a family of extremely religious Orthodox Jews. The outside world is shunned by her community. Women are expected to marry young, have many children, and rely upon their husbands for financial support. G is a strikingly beautiful woman with long, curly red hair. Though she is just twenty-four years old, her family believes that G is "over the hill." And perhaps she is. It will be extremely difficult for G to find an Orthodox man willing to marry such an "untraditional" Orthodox woman. G has already broken many mores within the community. While her family was surprised when she decided to attend a local community college, they were beside themselves with grief and anger when she eventually informed them that she was going to Harvard. In fact, her parents invited a rabbi to their home to talk G out of the decision, who explained that she would go to hell should she attend a secular college such as Harvard. She was completely alone, both financially and emotionally. Fortunately, over the years, her family has adjusted to G's "radical" lifestyle. I suppose that after going to Harvard, deciding to attend medical school wasn't all that traumatic. While her family seems to be coping well, G is now experiencing an identity crisis of sorts, as she is struggling to integrate Orthodox and secular values. Reflecting on G's story, it seems ironic that in any middleclass, secular household, G's intelligence and accomplishments would be commended, but that within Orthodox society she was ostracized.

And then there is S. He is a fourth-year stud, onetime marathon runner, sexy guitar player, and master chef who broke my heart earlier this year. One snowy December evening, he invited me over for a romantic dinner at his apartment. After shopping for the proper ingredients, we proceeded to cook a stir-fry masterpiece that was more an aphrodisiac than a dinner—a hot, bubbling combination of chicken, beef, water chestnuts, snow pea pods, carrots, baby corn, mushrooms, broccoli, and strange-looking peppers in a fantastic sauce of unknown origin. It was drippingly delicious, just like a scene out of *Like Water for Chocolate*. That night, we danced to K.D. Lang, made out, and spent a few glorious hours lying around in bed. Once he took off his glasses, I was a goner. Not to mention the things he said to me that night . . . For instance, "I'd be lying if I said I didn't want to make love to you, but wanting to do something isn't the same thing as having an expectation."

I replied, "I want to be in love with the next person I sleep with."

"Maybe you'll fall in love with me."

"Maybe I will."

I suppose it wasn't meant to be, as S ended things about a week later. I still don't understand the whole story behind this turn of events, but apparently, he had recently broken up with a serious girlfriend before we met. From what he later told me over tears and a cup of hot chocolate, I came to understand that fear of commitment had caused him to leave this woman. "She asked me where our relationship was going," he explained, "because I was going to leave for my residency at the end of the year. She didn't want to wait around for me if I wasn't willing to commit." After some soul-searching, S decided that he had left the relationship too hastily and wanted to give it another try.

As much as I wanted to hate him, I was unable to do so; S was much too confused to inspire hatred. In fact, I ended up wanting to befriend him more than anything else. In trying to sort out his emotions, S mentioned that he had suffered a difficult childhood. At an early age, his father abandoned the family to return to Pakistan (his native land), leaving the mother alone to raise S and his three siblings. The family hasn't heard from or seen the father since. S believes that he decided to return to his previous relationship, in part, because he didn't want to make the same mistake as his father, namely running away from a stable relationship in psychologically trying times.

By now, the reader might be thinking that all medical students are a product of secret, sordid, and horrific histories. That is just not the case. I know of at least two people who had "normal" childhood experiences and are genuinely interested in medicine. Well, not quite. One individual, B, has always wanted to be a pediatrician. The other "normal" person, L, maintains that she "came to medical school by default" because she couldn't think of anything better to do after college. For her and myself, medical school has served the important purpose of providing us with a sense of direction during a time when the "real world" seems completely directionless for college graduates. I suppose that my answer to R's original question isn't really that far off.

Due to my newfound, antiacademic attitude, I have done everything in my power to pretend that I am not actually a medical student. In fact, I have attempted to recapture that last year of college, which I gave up by accelerating. For instance, I've taken up long-distance running again, almost to an excessive degree. During my senior year in college, I was too busy taking classes and dealing with a rocky relationship to continue running, as I had done throughout high school. To make up for this, I have been running to Central Park almost every afternoon since school began. Luckily, about 25 percent of my class is as obsessed with running as I am; I never have trouble finding someone to drag down to the park. However, I did have a bit of trouble convincing my classmates to race with me in a half-marathon that took place in Brooklyn. While no one from the first-year class (except myself) signed up, two individuals from the second-year class were brave enough to endure the tortuous ordeal. We all crossed the finish line, a wonderful feeling. Unfortunately, I had difficulty walking for about a week afterward.

In addition to my running goals, I've started to pursue my desire to become a professional nightclub singer. Unfortunately, I really don't have the voice to sing professionally. The other day, I found a note from my roommate politely asking me not to sing so loudly in the bathroom. While this was a bit discouraging, I decided to take to the stage anyway. The perfect opportunity arose when a student group sponsored a "coffee house," an evening of singing, piano playing, poetry reading, stupid pet tricks, and son on performed by medical students. I was in heaven. An open microphone and the chance to display my hidden "talent." For what more could I ask? I found a friend with similar musical tastes who played the guitar, and we performed the Indigo Girls' song "Watershed." Even though no one came running to me after the show with a record contract, I was flying higher than an LSD addict for about a week. What really made the evening special was the fact that many of our classmates came to hear us perform, and they lavished us with compliments afterward. Never have I lived in a more supportive environment. The warm relationships that I have developed with my classmates/colleagues have more than made up for the academic hell of medical school.

Perhaps my experiences in gross anatomy best illustrate this dichotomy. During the first two quarters of school, gross anatomy was the bane of my existence. I despised changing into my dirty, smelly scrubs; performing tedious dissections which yielded few tangible results; crowding around dissection tables that I couldn't see because I'm too short; sliding around on the floor, which was always covered with phenol and other unidentifiable, oily substances; and being hit on by male fourth-year teaching assistants who thought they were God's gift to the human race, especially women. Without my three anatomy partners, I would not have survived. To make our situation bearable, we whiled away the hours by gossiping about anything and everything. We served as one another's personal psychiatrists. We talked about intimate details of our relationships that we wouldn't discuss with even our closest friends. There is something about communing over a dead body that compels one to reveal their inner soul. By the end of the second quarter, we spent most of our time talking, rather than dissecting. I remember one afternoon in particular. Out of the blue, M told us that over the weekend he had been sexually assaulted by a stranger on a bus. We were the first people he told, and he seemed quite shaken. That evening, L and I brought candy and cookies to M's room to cheer him up. The four of us, M, A, L, and myself have remained close since gross anatomy ended a few months ago. Next year, M and A are living together, and the same goes for L and me. I believe that these relationships are some of the strongest that we have developed thus far.

While L and I both take a pessimistic view of the factors which brought us to medical school, we are nevertheless optimistic about the future. Even though we detest sitting through unintelligible, medically irrelevant classes, which invariably put half the class to sleep (biostatistics, for example), we realize that the torture is temporary. Both of us are looking forward to our third year, the hospital "rotation" year, in which we actually get to work with patients. Already, our few experiences with patients have been surprisingly satisfying. L fell in love with working in the emergency room, where she served as a patient advocate. I enjoyed our psychiatry course, in which students interviewed patients from New York Hospital's psychiatric ward. That is, I enjoyed it most of the time. Unfortunately, the last time I interviewed a patient, he had a seizure right in the middle of the interview. Never have I felt so helpless and paralyzed! As much as I knew about histology and endocrinology from my textbooks, I could do nothing medically for this patient. Luckily, the resident came running in to try to revive him. When our class left the room, the patient was still out cold. A few weeks ago, I experienced a similar feeling when I witnessed a bloody rollerblading accident in Central Park. Skating down a hill fairly quickly, a young girl lost her balance and slammed her face against the asphalt. As she screamed for help, blood streaming out of her mouth, I knew that there was nothing I could do. I'm looking forward to the day when I won't feel so useless. Currently, I cringe when my relatives and nonmedical friends ask for advice, serious or not, about their medical problems. Perhaps my desire to feel competent has compelled me to remain in medical school thus far.

From these experiences, I've concluded that one probably does not start to become a "doctor" until third year, when patient care actually begins. On the other hand, my classmates and I are already becoming "professionalized." Each week when we don our white coats before psychiatry class, we assume a more responsible, cautious attitude. This change is brought about, in part, because the patients treat us as though we are doctors. Scary. If only they could see us getting drunk on Thursday nights at the local bar. That would probably take some of the mystique away from the profession. Recently, I was quite disheartened by a *New York Times* editorial which stated that medical students become clones of one another in the medical socialization process. Contrary to popular belief, medical students are not paper dolls. L is still wearing her Birkenstocks to class, and I'm still sporting my twenty-year-old cutoff jeans (though if they acquire any more holes, I'll probably be arrested for indecent exposure). Furthermore, though we all share a common drive to reach our goals, our histories, motivations, and approaches to survival are richly varied. While I hold onto my sanity by doing everything other than medical school, B maintains his composure by studying like a maniac and staying two weeks ahead of every class. Some of us have always wanted to become doctors and are fulfilling a lifelong dream, while others are just confused, trying to figure out how they got here in the first place. Despite these differences, we share the hope that we've made the right decision and that things will somehow work out in the end. After all, if it turns out that medicine isn't the right career for me, there's always nightclub singing. Maybe.

Allison Beitel
Cornell University Medical College
Class of 1997

BROKEN HEARTS

Back in medical school, when I wrote "Trapped on the First-Year Roller Coaster" for the book *Becoming Doctors*, I was young, self-centered, and rebellious, living in New York City for the first time, second guessing my decision to become a physician. Over the course of the past twenty-five years, my life has changed dramatically. In addition to becoming a wife and mother, I successfully completed medical school, residency, and a pediatric emergency medicine fellowship. For the past sixteen years, I have worked in the trenches as a general pediatrician, overseeing the care of sick and well children at all stages of development.

Although I initially doubted my career choice, the job has been fulfilling in ways that I could not have appreciated in my twenties. On a global scale, for example, pediatricians provide lifesaving vaccines to the youngest members of our society. As a medical student, I didn't spend time pondering the public health benefits of vaccinating children, but performing this service over the years has been good for my soul. On an individual level, the care I've provided to patients and families has also been gratifying. Looking back on my career, the most memorable patients I encountered were those who were presented with life-threatening conditions, unbeknownst to the parents, and the cases bear striking similarities.

During my first week on the job as a general pediatrician in private practice, I encountered a family with a three-day-old baby needing a weight check. A quick chart review confirmed the infant had lost more than 10 percent of her birth weight. When I entered the room, she was lying quietly on the table, hardly moving her arms and legs. On exam, I was alarmed to discover a hyperdynamic precordium, and I asked the parents whether any cardiac problems had been detected in utero.

"Well, yes," said the mother, looking perplexed. "Our obstetrician told us something didn't look right on an ultrasound a few months ago; but everything seemed fine at the hospital after she was born."

"Did the baby have an echocardiogram before leaving the hospital?" I asked.

"No, but the residents examined her, and they said everything was okay."

Wondering if something significant had been missed with this child, I proceeded to check the baby's femoral pulses. Although the infant wasn't moving, I was unable to appreciate *any* femoral pulse.

Trying not to be an alarmist, I turned to the parents and said, "I'm sure everything is going to be fine, but it might be a good idea to see a cardiologist . . . today."

Several hours later, the baby was diagnosed with a critical aortic coarctation and admitted to the pediatric intensive care unit. Though her medical course has been rather complicated, I'm happy to report the infant has grown up to become a mostly healthy young woman whom I continue to care for on a regular basis.

More recently, a baby with a similar problem was presented for a routine weight check. At first glance, this infant looked extremely well. He was alert and active, with a healthy pink complexion. I was surprised, therefore, when I couldn't locate a femoral pulse. For about fifteen minutes, I tried altering the position of his hips and legs, thinking my physical exam skills must really be going down the tubes, but I still couldn't appreciate the pulse. Upon reviewing the baby's hospital chart, I realized the hospitalist hadn't been able to find one, either. Reassuringly, four-extremity blood pressures had been normal before discharge.

Because the baby looked so well, the parents were skeptical that the infant required an immediate evaluation. After a twenty-four-hour delay in care, while the parents tended a sick dog who was unfortunately dying at home, the baby was diagnosed with an aortic coarctation and promptly scheduled for surgery. I'm still kicking myself for allowing the next-day referral; in that short time period, the baby could have gone into shock. On this occasion, we all got lucky.

The third case of left-sided heart failure I encountered unfortunately didn't end well. A one-week-old baby came in for a weight check, and I noted that after a brief period of weight gain, she had lost more than 10 percent of her birth weight. On exam, the baby seemed listless, lying on the exam table, barely moving—similar to the first child with the aortic coarctation.

While I was able to palpate her femoral pulses, they seemed weaker than normal, and I started to worry about the heart. On auscultation, I detected a murmur that hadn't been present a few days earlier. Although I didn't know exactly what was wrong with the baby, I was worried about a possible coarctation. After some initial resistance and haranguing, the family agreed to return to the hospital, where the baby was evaluated by pediatric cardiology. Although the echocardiogram demonstrated normal anatomy, the left ventricular function was markedly impaired. During an evaluation in the cardiac catheterization lab, the situation deteriorated. The baby coded, underwent an extensive resuscitation, and was eventually placed on ECMO. Head imaging in the aftermath demonstrated significant brain damage, and the family chose to withdraw life support. Postmortem testing identified a common infection, one that is normally harmless in children, as the cause of death: coxsackie virus.

During the course of the baby's illness, I sat with the family in the hospital, hugged the devastated parents, and offered emotional support. As traumatic as these events were for all of us, the sun kept rising and life pressed onward. Several years later, the family has two new healthy children—a twin boy and girl who were conceived after several rounds of IVF, and I am grateful to be their provider.

Given the choice, would I still choose to become a pediatrician if I could go back in time, knowing what I know now? Wholeheartedly the answer is yes. While I'm unable to fix every medical problem that comes my way, pediatrics has allowed me to build a career based upon the central principle of helping others, and I can't think of a better way to live.

Allison Beitel, M.D.
Pediatrics

SOUL SURVIVOR

How can I best describe the odor of a preserved cadaver? Sushi, pickles, lox, jerky, Spam, tuna, and chicken. Such odors sketch only the faintest outline of this aroma. For this smell is far stranger and subtler than any I have inhaled before—familiar, yet exotic; unforgettable, yet inexpressible. It is a mix of flesh and fluid, glycerol and formaldehyde. It is the body's decay chemically frozen in time. When the doors to our dissecting room are opened, it is this bizarre odor which pours forth to welcome our visitors. The ancient Greeks believed that a vital breath of *pneuma* departed from the body of the deceased. Perhaps the strong odor of our laboratory shares in this preternatural component. One first must inhale this gas, this *pneuma*, these "spirits" of the dead, before one can dissect the bodies from which they have escaped. I try to breathe deeply, fully, and heavily throughout each and every human dissection I perform.

I am a first-year medical student, and human dissection is my first-year rite of passage. Our required course in human anatomy continues this aged tradition of Hippocrates and others by initiating us into the medical rituals of gross anatomical human dissection. Immediately following our initial class lecture, each of us receives a key to the Laboratory of Human Anatomy, a tour of the facilities, and an introduction to the "specimens" with which we will become increasingly "familiar" throughout the term. The laboratory has three main classrooms, and each possesses not just the usual blackboards, chalk, tables, and chairs, but also scalpels, bone saws, scissors, probes, tweezers, suction pumps, disinfectant, sinks, and of course, several rows of large dissecting tables. In the middle of one such table, beneath the focus of a pair of bright halogen lamps, the "specimen" for my dissection lies sealed within a blue vinyl body bag.

I pull away the large black zippers and roll the bag flaps over to the side. It is the first time I have ever seen a dead human body. The head, hands, and feet of the corpse are covered with sock-like cotton bags—as if the cadaver somehow decided to wear mittens, booties, and a thick ski mask. Each of these coverings is to be removed only when its respective region is to be dissected. This occlusion of the hands, feet, and face, all distinctly human features, is intended to dehumanize the "specimens," thus giving us students time to adjust to the more psychologically jarring aspects of bodily dissection. Yet the modesty of each body is left completely unshielded, with the penis fully exposed on each male cadaver and the vagina and breasts similarly revealed on each female. I remember warnings concerning our own sexuality and how it might be challenged by the discipline of human dissection. But most cadavers are seventy to ninety years old, and so, contrary to any suppressed preadolescent fantasies, I am denied the delicate task of dissecting some young plasticene poster model. My cadaver is markedly older, more flaccid, and more atrophied. He was an eighty-year-old gentleman who died of complications due to prostate cancer.

"Nice to meet you, sir." It is a strange urge, but it seemed natural at the time. My first response on meeting this man's body is to reach forward and shake his hand. It is the first time I have ever touched dead human flesh. Dead skin looks very much alive. It has a color which seems quite normal, perhaps a bit pallid, and a texture which seems quite typical, with hair, freckles, moles, and scars all relatively intact. But dead skin feels nothing at all like the living. It is cold, hard, and rigid. As I reach forward to shake the hand of my cadaver, the musculature resists my gesture. It is compressed, frozen in place by *rigor mortis*. Living tissue generates a special sugar that allows the fibers of each muscle to slide past one another. Upon death, this sugary "oil of life" recedes from the muscles, and so the limbs thus become locked in *rigor mortis*, rusted tight like the Tin Man of Oz. Dorothy was able to find a magic can of oil with which to revive the Tin Man, but no known can of oil will revive this gentleman's body, and clearly, none was able to prevent his death. However, the study of human anatomy does give us a foundation upon which to begin the search.

It appears as though every structure in the human body, no matter how small, no matter how seemingly insignificant, necessarily has serious clinical significance. We ask our professors, "Do we need to know this for the exam?" and the response is, as always, "My dear students, you should seek to be encyclopedic." I have been told that most doctors forget about 90 percent of the anatomy they learn in medical school, but the 10 percent most do remember is used 90 percent of the time. Such statistics comfort me as I struggle with my notes, diagrams, and textbooks late through the night and on into the early morning.

I approach my study of human anatomy with what is for me an unprecedented fervor. I no longer am studying just for my own personal pleasure, at my own leisurely pace, but I now have an obligation, a duty, and a responsibility to study as forcefully, copiously, and rigorously as I possibly can. A fellow human being has donated his body so that I may have the privilege of human dissection. I thus have learned more about this person than he perhaps ever could have learned about himself. I have thoroughly inspected his body— his insides, his outsides, and the structures in between; the foundations from his birth; the scaffoldings of his life; and the final cracks, breaks, and ruptures which tumbled him to his death.

Although his body and I have become intimate friends, his name remains a mystery to me. All cadaver donations are strictly anonymous, and so I probably never will learn this name. It is a popular custom among my classmates to cope with the stress of human dissection by "naming" their cadavers. I rebelliously cope by refusing to name mine, referring to him only as "the gentleman." My cadaver once was alive; he had a mother, a father, perhaps a wife, maybe a child, and most certainly, a name. He had a name in life, so who am I to rename him in death? Perhaps, one day, in whatever may lie beyond, we will have an opportunity to meet, his soul and mine. If so, I will greet him warmly, thank him ardently, commend him for his generous gift, and then perhaps, finally get a chance to ask him for his name.

One month into the term, we students have spent about twelve hours a week, almost fifty hours in total, surrounded by cadavers, skeletons, and various other human body parts of all shapes and sizes. It all seems so normal now. When we first arrived in the dissecting classrooms, we were timid, gentle, and slow; we would meekly touch the cadavers, poke them cautiously with our tools, double gloves over each hand, and then, after the dissection, run to the sink and wash ourselves thoroughly under scalding water with pitchers of disinfectant. It would be several hours before any of us recovered emotionally enough to eat, and many students felt further compelled to take long showers immediately afterward to obliterate that pervasive odor of preserved cadaver. But the human ability to adapt is incredible—our class has become perhaps far too familiar with this environment. After four weeks of daily dissections, we run to the room following each lecture, quickly throw on a pair of gloves and perhaps a loose smock, boldly rip open the cadavers, and dive in with tools and hands and fingers, pushing and pulling, tugging and tossing body parts out across the table. Finally, after a brisk rinse of hands in the sink, we are off to the supper table, hungry for a full dinner.

I am in the anatomy lab so much that I give out the phone number to my friends and family. They phone me, and I take the call, balancing the phone between my shoulder and my ear, both gloved hands just having been removed from the guts of a cadaver, every finger still dripping and glistening with miscellaneous human ooze. Then, perhaps later, I will be at home, talking to my mother on the telephone, lying on my pillow and playfully running my fingers through the grooves of a real human skull from the set of bones each of us was given for take-home study. But beneath this thin veneer of equanimity lies a thicker layer of amazement. Our anatomy professors seem to take an almost macabre pleasure in listing for us—with graphic photographs—the innumerable things which can, and do, go wrong with the human body. There are so many diseases, disorders, and defects! I no longer can see how anyone is ever born at all, or ever eats, sleeps, walks, and grows. It now appears miraculous to me that any of us can move a muscle, breathe a breath, think a thought, or dream a dream.

Anatomy class has stolen from me this mortal sight. I no longer see people as I once did. My vision of my fellow human beings has been blinded by my knowledge of their dissection. I used to look at a person the way one might look at a building, as just being there, existing. Now, I look at each part of that person and each brick in that building, and within my mind, I take the structure apart and put it back together, again and again, over and over and over. My eyes continually and uncontrollably dissect each and every person I meet. My gaze cuts through the surface of their humanity and directly into the core of their flesh.

Some prefer to dismiss this flesh as being irrelevant, distinctly separable from the soul. But I have come to appreciate the flesh as an integral part of the reality of each person's existence. We may agree that flesh is just the clothing of the soul, but it is a cloth which can never be removed. No one gets to choose it for themselves, and it can never be returned, refunded, or exchanged. It tears easily, it mends poorly, and it is doomed to decay and decompose. Yet flesh provides the only known cloth for the soul, and as such, it is necessarily a cloth of tremendous beauty, miraculous intricacy, and passionate wonder. To be a doctor, then, is to have the privilege of tailoring this tapestry, mending the rips, sewing the tears, cleansing the seams, and dusting the folds.

I spent this evening in the dissecting lab, fishing out with my fingers the last remnants of blood from our cadaver's heart. This was the very blood which settled motionlessly when his heart stopped beating and then coagulated within the still vessels of his body. I have had to cut out this human heart and place it within my hands. It is a thick, muscular pump, with rough walls that belie the intricacy and delicacy of the cellular components within. This machine pumped continuously throughout this man's life, from before his birth and until his death, a rhythm of sixty beats per minute, more or less, with little tolerance for error or deviation.

I place his heart next to his brain upon the table. The nerve cells within the living brain constantly send out extensions to communicate with one another, and these biological wires continually move, reform, rotate, and reconnect, all over the course of a lifetime in response to the external environment, an environment which they in turn can affect, thus affecting themselves. The brain boasts this fine, recursive cellular structure that takes a lifetime to complete, and so if ever a shadow of this man's soul remains upon the material plane, I would guess it to be within his brain. But I have cut open his brain and searched. There is no shining gem within, no preternatural conduit for a soul to enter our world.

I look back to the heart. I look again to the brain. I return to my cadaver and stare into his lifeless eyes. Is this all there is?

If flesh is considered just the clothing of the soul, then where lies the soul itself? Where? Within which organ of the body does the soul reside? From ancient times to the present, the soul has been placed variously in the heart, the brain, the diaphragm, the belly, the eyes, the cerebellum, and the cerebral ventricles. Some even suggest the soul is to be found nowhere at all. Is the soul wherever you look for it? Is the soul wherever you find it?

If we could somehow exhaust the seemingly inexhaustible possibilities and so conclude that no soul exists, then the body becomes nothing less than the sole survivor. If we should eventually discover a secret hiding place for the soul and so conclude that the soul exists, then the body becomes nothing more than the soul's survivor. In either case, the human body ever and always would remain the human body. And it is really quite a lot for us medical students to study, perhaps more than enough. At least, for now.

Adam Strassberg
Stanford University School of Medicine
Class of 1998

FISH GONE, GOING FISHING

It was another day in the office, seemingly like any other. I finished work as usual, turned off the lights as usual, and closed the door as usual, but then, unusually, I slid my name plate from its holder down into my black briefcase. It was my last day in the office, and suddenly, just like that, I was retired.

The next morning, a portable shredder truck came and shredded away twenty years of patient files in under twenty minutes. And just like that, I was done. I had been a psychiatrist in private practice for twenty years in Silicon Valley. I completed my medical degree at nearby Stanford University, next my psychiatric training there as well. I married, bought a home, raised children, and, for the next twenty years, rented the same small office only a few blocks away from all of it.

I had few emotions the next few days, but a week later, after I rehomed my two prized big fancy goldfish and gave away my large office fish tank, I cried for many, many hours. I sat upon the bench in the atrium of my waiting room. It was a sunny day with fluffy white clouds circling the sky. I looked over at my empty door and empty office, took out my handkerchief, and began a tremendous session of tearful abreaction. I wept.

Elisabeth Kubler-Ross identified five stages of grief: denial, anger, depression, bargaining, and finally acceptance. The stages are not really stages, as they are neither linear nor ordinal, but they do seem to summarize the various parts of the grieving process. Her model originally was developed to describe how terminally ill patients cope with the dying process, but it later was expanded to include how people cope with most any sort of loss. In my case, the loss of a professional

140

role identity. I was a practicing psychiatrist. The loss does not have to be involuntary; it can be volitional; it can be a measured choice. But a loss is still a loss. And thus now, by choice, I am no longer a practicing psychiatrist.

And I no longer have my two fish buddies. "Siggy" and "Carl" had been my inveterate vertebrate companions through two decades of outpatient psychotherapy and psychopharmacology. They were my only office staff. They were my resident residents, and I was their attentive attending. I fed them daily, changed their filter tank cartridge monthly, and added fresh water to their fifty-five-gallon tank whenever it evaporated by a bucket or so.

Originally, they were two small oranda fantail goldfish, one orange, one calico (white with blue and black spots), each less than a quarter in length. Over the decades, they grew to the length of a full dollar bill and the girth of a half dollar coin. I named them—"Siggy" was the orange one, "Carl," the calico one. They hovered there together, silent gentle witnesses, nobly present at each and every clinical visit over the years. They were the ideal co-therapists, paragons of perfection from a psychodynamic perspective. Excellent eye contact, active listening, reactive expressivity, and securely attached, yet strictly forbidden from directly interacting with a patient by an impenetrable glass wall. Per custom, neither they nor I ever physically touched a patient in my office.

Over the decades, my two goldfish have listened to strangers confess marital infidelities, monetary fraud, sexual peccadilloes, religious crises, and moral dilemmas. They have seen me aid and comfort and often cure these and other patients who variably hear voices, see visions, cannot sleep, repeat involuntary rituals, fight urges to cut or burn themselves, write suicide notes, yield to overwhelming sadness, run from anxieties, abuse substances, hide from traumatic memories, and otherwise act and react to the vast diversity of human harm and dysfunction chronicled in the 157 diagnoses within the latest edition of the *Diagnostics and Statistical Manual of Mental Disorders.*

Siggy and Carl have witnessed thousands of hours of psychotherapy sessions and hundreds of hours of medication management visits. I often have imagined what these two goldfish might have been saying to each other while I worked. "Interesting choice of his to use a nonverbal referent just there." "Wow, that is some serious projective identification." "Note the guarded body language when she talks about her mother."

"That's a bold use of paradox." "How can he not interpret that reaction formation?" "Wow, that's a high dose of antipsychotic. I hope he remembers to check the hemoglobin A1c." "Nice use of symptom magnification to expose his denial." "This one clearly needs a referral for TMS or ECT."

I wonder what their famous namesakes would have to say about them. Siggy is named after Sigmund Freud. The father of psychiatry did not have much to say about fish specifically, but he did find water symbolic. It represents birth and rebirth. One plunges into water or climbs out of it, rescues someone from water or gets rescued. It is a motherlike relationship, as literally we are all born from the waters of our mothers' wombs. For patients, perhaps the process of therapy is akin to a process of rebirth. They are reborn into very different people whence they began. Carl is named after Carl Jung. To this great mythologist, water symbolized the unconscious. One can see the surface of water but cannot easily see into its depths. Fish become symbols to describe psychic experiences that suddenly dart out of the unconscious. Notably then, a fish tank literally reveals these depths, and particularly those fish beneath the water's surface, much as psychotherapy metaphorically reveals those depths, and particularly those psychic experiences "darting out" beneath the subconscious's surface.

My use of a large fish tank in my office, however, had much less to do with psychodynamic psychotherapy and considerably more to do with behaviorism. Fish make me happy. My earliest memory is of rocking in a chair in my father's arms, mesmerized by the large fish tank in our home. Soothed by the steady vibrations of innumerable pumps and siphons, I fell asleep nightly to a lullaby of air bubbles, running water, humming machinery, and, of course, my daddy's heartbeat. Fish make me feel safe. The tank connects me to my father's spirit. Later in my childhood, our dentist installed an enormous wall tank to relax and distract his patients. It worked almost too well. We actually wanted to visit the dentist, the reward of viewing his majestic tank outweighing the punishment from the dental procedures. I surmised that a large fish tank might have the same effect upon my therapy patients and so purchased one the day I signed my lease. I considered it a crucial piece of office equipment, and peer-reviewed academic studies later emerged to support this suspicion.

In a 2015 study published in the journal *Environment and Behavior*, Dr. Deborah Cracknell and her colleagues studied the psychological effects of watching fish in an aquarium. They found significant reductions in heart rate and blood pressure within the first five minutes of viewing. Mood improved. As the duration of exposure increased, the subjects became more positive and calmer. This fits with the obvious—nature makes people happy. E.O. Wilson called it his *biophilia hypothesis*—human beings have an innate instinct to connect emotionally with the natural world. It is now all part of a branch of psychology dubbed "ecopsychology," the study of the relationship between human beings and the natural world through ecological and psychological principles. For me, as a part of my clinical practice, it represents a commitment to bringing as much of the natural world as possible into my therapy office—potted plants, fish tanks, a fireplace, candles, etc.—whenever and wherever possible. Nature is restorative and alleviates human stress and fatigue. My goldfish and their fish tank were tools to do just that.

And so Siggy and Carlworked daily beside me, humbly and nobly, with dedication and devotion for nearly two decades of service. The lifespan of goldfish is reported to range from five to fifty years, but their true lifespan may be unknowable. Like many fish, fantail oranda goldfish may share a resistance to biological aging. *Senescence*, the scientific term for biological aging, is the property of a life form wherein its probability of dying increases each year of life. Some fish, turtles, and other vertebrates seem to have essentially negligible senescence. They die from predation, accidents, and disease, but do not seem to otherwise age cellularly. I netted my two prized goldfish and gently transferred each into separate plastic bags filled by half with tank water. I closed each bag rapidly to catch the air, tied it taut with a rubber band, and then placed them together into a large bucket. I blew a kiss and said my last goodbyes to Siggy and Carl. A dear friend volunteered to rehome them in his new tank. He took the bucket from me and loaded them into his car. Perhaps they will swim another twenty years in this next aquarium, perhaps longer. I watched the car drive away and then returned to sit upon the bench in the waiting area of my office. I was sad. I was tired. These beloved fish may have negligible senescence, but not so human psychiatrists. Not so me.

I am aging. I am growing old.

I forget things now. "Age-related cognitive decline" is not so much a diagnosis as a description applicable to most of us by our late forties. I occasionally mistake the names of drugs and dosages; I recheck myself obsessively, like most physicians. Nobody knows—no mistakes, no consequences, yet—but I know. I am at 90 percent capacity of my thirty-year-old self. When will it be 80 percent? Seventy percent? This common condition worsens as the day progresses. One evening last summer, both my wife and I entered the same room from opposite doors, and neither of us could remember why we were there. A good laugh, but also a good epiphany. It was time.

I never thought I would retire. In my thirties, with a new practice, I was excited each year to get several new patients from the latest local octogenarian psychiatrist who literally died in the chair. Most psychiatrists never retire, and I too always believed that I would work until I died. The practice is so very rewarding. Between medications and psychotherapies, we are able to help most patients improve and recover. Also, psychiatry is much more an art than a science, and the actual drugs and treatments advance very slowly, so it is very easy to stay current—unlike my agemates in engineering, for example, where exponential advances typically force them to either move up to management or move out to an early ageist forced retirement.

I think back to my thirties. Those years were so very generative between me and friends and neighbors; it was all about getting married and making children, growing, and building—homes, careers, wealth, and bounty. But the forties were ever so much more tenuous, so fearful. It was all about divorce, cancer, heart disease, death, and destruction all around us, with survivor guilt for those of us who avoided these mid-life catastrophes. When I was forty-four, my father died. By forty-seven, I had lost two similarly aged friends, one to cancer, another to heart disease.

The fantasy of literally dying in the chair while working as an ancient psychiatrist gave way to the reality of, well, dying. My wife retired a few years back, our children flew off to college, and we became empty nesters. I knew it was time. If you are lucky enough to be able to retire, you really should retire as soon as you can. You sort of owe it to yourself and to everyone else to do so humbly and quietly. Oldness must make way for newness. But can oldness beget newness? If I retire by age fifty, I can do a whole other thing, be a whole other person, and have a third other act in my later life.

And so, I return home to our empty nest, kiss my wife, and place my briefcase on the bench, with my nameplate still inside. My wife has been busy too today, planning the furniture and finishings for our new cozy cottage by the river. We move next month. Downsizing and simplifying. Perhaps a small bowl with some tiny goldfish would fit nicely there. Or perhaps the river nearby will have all the fish I need.

Years ago, I became a doctor. I was a doctor. Now I will unbecome a doctor.

And soon I can be just me.

Adam Strassberg, M.D.
Psychiatry

LEARNING TO LISTEN

Mrs. R was dying of grossly metastatic ovarian cancer. She was bedridden and very ill. It was mid-August, and I was finishing my second week as a third-year medical student. My head was whirling with all the facts I had learned in the past fortnight. It felt as though I had learned more in the last thirteen days than I had during the whole twelve months of the second year. But it was Saturday, and after I had finished rounds, I had a whole day-and-a-half off. It was a bright summer's day outside, and I had intended to get my progress notes done quickly and leave to enjoy my rare free time. However, when I spoke to Mrs. R that morning, I knew that she was becoming more and more depressed and despondent. She had repeatedly refused a psychiatry consult, and I had actually entertained the thought of putting her on antidepressants anyway. I knew that that was not the answer for her, but I felt frustrated. As I wrote my notes and discussed this problem with my resident, I realized that this would haunt me until Monday morning. I did not want to be depressed all weekend about Mrs. R's depression, so I decided to go back and talk to her once I had finished my work.

It was now 11 AM, and I had an out-of-town guest waiting for me and my deluxe tour of New York City. I put my friend out of my mind and sat down with Mrs. R. I expressed my concern for her and asked her if there was anything I could do. She laughed—how could a healthy young woman like me know what she was going through? I did not move. After it became clear that I wasn't going anywhere, she opened up to me. She explained that she had worked all her life, and that lying in bed all day with others bringing her food and medication made her feel totally useless and helpless. I had no idea how to respond and wished that I had picked psychiatry as my first rotation instead of medicine. But deep down, I knew that what

I said was much less important than the simple fact that I was there to listen; therefore, I stayed silent until she was completely finished. Despite my feeling at a total loss for words, I responded as if she were a friend of mine and simply expressed my sympathy. I knew that there was nothing I could do to make her cancer go away. There was nothing I could do to help her walk again. Everything I did—the blood draws, the chemotherapy orders, the daily physicals, and progress notes—was really a weak attempt to stave off the inevitable. Everybody, from Mrs. R herself to the hem/onc attending, knew that she would die soon. I felt helpless. Yet as I sat there, doing my best to keep my mouth shut so that she could talk (and trying to say the right things when I was brave enough to speak), I realized that that was all I could offer her, but it was the most anyone could offer her. She didn't want a psychiatrist because she felt that only crazy people saw psychiatrists. That did not mean that she did not need someone to talk to. As I left the floor an hour-and-a-half later, very late to meet my friend, I realized that I had learned the first really important thing so far in my third year. Lists of differentials and drug dosages would come and go, but the idea of just listening would stay.

As a medical student, I often have the time when I am on the floor to just be with my patients. I know that that luxury will disappear the moment I start my internship. For now, I will enjoy it while I can. Although I had been motivated by the selfish impulse of not wanting to worry about Mrs. R all weekend, the results were much greater than the motivation. I understood the things I could do to help her, such as asking physical therapy to assist her into a wheelchair and getting her involved in some activities. She actually thanked me for listening when I returned on Monday; I didn't need the thanks because in so many ways, she helped me much more than I helped her.

We are taught things in medical school, but rarely are we given the opportunity to learn more about our patients than their biological malfunctioning. First and second years are packed full of biochemical pathways, drug metabolism, and pathophysiology of diseases. At the end of second year, I could explain all about the antibodies involved with lupus, but I could not begin to describe what having the disease is like for the patient. We are never taught what it really means to have one of the diseases we study; yet this is something that is vitally important to understand in order to be an effective doctor. There is an elective offered to second-year students at my medical school that tries to teach some of this. Students are paired up with patients who do not have visitors to spend time with them every day while they are in the hospital. This is a very popular elective, and I did not get a place in it last year. In retrospect, that seems absurd—I know that there are many patients, both adults and children, who could use a regular visitor while hospitalized. This sort of program should be open to all who want it at all medical schools.

If we do not take the time to learn to listen while we are medical students, we will never learn to listen when we are doctors.

Louise C. Greenspan
Cornell University Medical College
Class of 1995

Just Like Me

I remember an experience I had in medical school just over twenty-five years ago. I was on my third-year medicine clerkship, in the first month of my first clinical rotation. There was a Russian lady—I swore I'd never forget her name, and I haven't. She was dying of ovarian cancer, obstructed with stool. I cried at her plight. My attending physician pulled me aside; I thought I was going to be told off for being "overemotional."

Now, in those days, this was an old-fashioned, traditional school with a picture of King George III in the lobby, and it was staffed mostly by white men in their fifties to sixties with "Jr." or "III" after their name (or so it seemed to me). This attending physician was young but still a WASP and a male. He pulled me to a quiet part of the hallway and looked at me sternly and said (in my memory, he pointed his finger at me), "Don't *ever* forget this moment. Hold on to the way you feel today, and you will be a great doctor." This made me cry more and still brings tears to my eyes to this day. I felt that this attending physician heard me, understood me. He truly listened to me and allowed me to listen to my patient.

I have had too much experience since, being a physician as well as a patient. I've seen plenty of specialists. All very smart, no doubt. But the best of them are compassionate; I can see they care. They have also taught me how to take care of myself. But how many listened, how many understood what being a patient really feels like? How many had an attending physician pull them aside as an MS3 and let them cry?

How can I harness my twenty-four-year-old self and always remember, even at 2 AM, that the person on the other end of the call center advice call is a scared, worried parent, no matter how silly their question seems to me? How can I remind myself to see the person there? It's easy with my patients—they are kids. But the baggage that brings them—their

149

parents. . . . I need to get back to remembering that at times, we are all scared and worried and need some support and compassion. Just like me.

How many times since medical school have I sat in a waiting room reviewing the list of all the items I need to cover with my physician, afraid that I might forget something important, but also not wanting to waste their time? Then I return to my own clinic and see a parent with a spiral notebook and a long list of questions, and I take a deep breath and encourage them to ask every single one. Because they don't know what is important and what is not. Just like me.

How many times have I listened to a physician go over the pros and cons of a new treatment, and, knowing those rare side effects, I ask about those? The risk of blindness may be less than 1/1,000, but that's too high for my comfort level. Then I head back to my office to an email from a parent who has looked on Dr. Google and is worried about the new medication I put their child on. Just like me.

How many times have I laid on a stretcher, waiting for a procedure or test, and suddenly felt so vulnerable? Just a thin gown and blanket covering me, as I think about what I am about to get done. Then I hear the staff nearby chatting about their weekends, or what they had for lunch, or sharing a meme and laughing. And at first, it makes me mad because it seems like they aren't being respectful. But then I realize that they may be stressed or worn out, and laughing with their colleagues keeps them going. Just like me.

How many times have I worked with a medical student, seen the curiosity in their eyes, the wonder, and the raw desire to just learn and help in any way they can? The innocence, the youth. I remember me at that stage, and I want to harness it.

They are just like me. Well, just like I was.

If we do not take the time to learn to listen while we are medical students, we will never learn to listen when we are doctors.

Louise C. Greenspan, M.D.
Endocrinology

MY DUTY

He has eaten many meals,
Yet he is still hungry.
They have felt the warmth of many suns,
Yet they are still cold.
She has been among many crowds,
Yet she is still alone.

Let us offer him our food,
So that he will know fulfillment.
Let us share with them our heart,
So that they will know warmth.
Let us bring her into our thoughts,
So that she will know friendship.

Par Bolina
University of Illinois College of Medicine at Chicago
Class of 1996

MEDICINE'S DILEMMA

During the Summer between my first and second year of medical school, while doing an ICU rotation at the John Radcliffe Hospital in Oxford, England, I wrote the preceding poem on the back of a postcard and sent it to my medical school roommate in the U.S. explaining what I thought becoming an M.D. meant to me. Now, a few decades later, I share my thoughts about being a physician and, at the end, ask you a few questions to learn what you think about the work we do.

Throughout our lives, countless times every day, we decide whether something is good or bad. Afterwards, we probably do not spend much time reflecting whether we were right or wrong. Perhaps under the pressure of time, we rely on these original decisions and instead focus our attention on new ideas and new choices. When we step into a new environment, a new school, or a new job, where we are unfamiliar with almost everything, we may struggle even more to sort right from wrong, good from bad, and therefore we often accept the choices and recommendations of others we hope we can trust. Such an approach likely works well and creates consensus and cohesion among the newly initiated and the seasoned veterans until we begin to doubt whether the group's decisions are good ideas worth trusting. Encountering this dilemma is never easy; yet how one responds profoundly impacts the individual and their future. Surprisingly, how the group responds has an equally profound impact on everyone's future.

Throughout the history of medicine, there have been countless moments of doubt when younger physicians must choose between acceptance and conformity versus rejection and experimentation. This choice is neither welcomed by the young physician nor understood by their peers and supervisors. Those few physicians who risk their reputations and careers to experiment have frequently contributed to the advancement of medicine.

In a profession where wrong decisions may result in serious harm or death, the gravitational force of conformity is especially strong. However, the practice of treating and receiving medical care is also further complicated by a remarkably broad reluctance to question what is right from wrong, good or bad by almost everyone involved. Across the globe, medical students, doctors, staff, healthcare executives, and patients hesitate to challenge our approach to basic healthcare delivery. Sadly, significant change usually occurs only after we inadvertently harm or kill many. This combination of a reluctance to recognize along with the steady pressure to conform is and has been medicine's dilemma for decades. Unless we rethink our approach to basic healthcare delivery, we will continue to live in a self-imposed age of darkness, lit only by moments of courage, kindness, and clarity.

In the 1840s, a Hungarian physician scientist, Dr. Ignaz Semmelweis, working in Vienna could not understand why the maternal mortality rate was so high in the clinic managed by medical students compared to the clinic where student midwives conducted the deliveries. Ultimately, he suspected that the medical students studying anatomy on corpses may have been carrying "cadaverous particles" on their unwashed hands, which later came in contact with the mothers during delivery, causing a harmful infection. After instituting a handwashing policy for the medical students, the maternal mortality dramatically reduced to near zero. Unfortunately, over the next decade, Dr. Semmelweis was unable to convince his peers to widely adopt handwashing. Without clear evidence or proof, his peers dismissed his observations, warnings, and recommendations regarding decaying organic matter. As a result, Dr. Semmelweis's career suffered, and ultimately, he died in a mental institution. A few years after his death, a French scientist, Louis Pasteur, confirmed the germ theory and later, a British surgeon, Dr. Joseph Lister, relying on their work, pioneered antiseptic surgery, saving countless lives.

Almost a hundred years later, a Yale physician scientist, Dr. Lawrence Weed, who primarily conducted microbial genetics research, would occasionally supervise medical students on their hospital rounds. He noted with frustration and alarm that the students struggled to understand the medical charts because the notes followed no pattern, were hard to read, and failed to clearly indicate what the patient was being treated for. Because he suspected a strong link between poor documentation and the risk of harm to the patients, he created and advocated for a novel structured way for all doctors to write patient notes. Over the next several decades he published and lectured on the benefits of such an approach as well as outlining the risks of continued poor documentation. Ultimately, the medical community relented and eventually accepted the SOAP note format. Today, throughout the world, medical students and doctors are taught to follow his method, and as a result, countless lives have been saved.

Like my fellow authors, few of us would have known of these stories and examples as we enjoyed the privilege of spending our twenties in medical school and residency learning to become doctors. Our focus was to learn and replicate as much as we could from our physician teachers, trusting they and the other instructors knew best. Our ability to precisely recall what we are taught was rewarded with good test scores, better options to select a specialty, and eventually, an opportunity to earn more throughout our career.

During residency, as we began to spend more time in the clinics, we realized that practicing medicine requires becoming an effective teacher, advisor, coach, and advocate who translates all the science, the latest studies, and probabilities into understandable options for each patient to consider. Over the years, we listened and learned about our patient's concerns and worries with the intent to make a meaningful impact in their life. With practice, feedback, and mentoring, we became better at this enjoyable but demanding vocation.

After years of learning and teaching, upon entering private practice in my thirties, I encountered a strange silence. Unlike my residency training, in private practice, few of my colleagues discussed cases, supervised students, or provided formal or informal feedback to each other. Equally surprising, perhaps for the first time ever, I alone decided how to manage my time. Initially, as I introduced myself to my colleagues, I tried to understand how to accomplish the very basics of being a doctor in private practice. Specifically, I wanted to know what should my priorities be; what should my work hours be; what type of patients should I see; what should I ask of nurses and staff versus do on my own; what are my goals; and how will I know if I'm doing well? It turns out that how a physician answers these basic questions likely influences the trajectory of their career more than almost anything else.

During this discovery phase, I realized two things about myself and my job. First, I genuinely enjoyed encountering a diversity of patients with an array of problems every day at work. Remarkably, for helping the patients with their problems, I not only earned their gratitude, but I was also very well compensated. Secondly, in order to both excel at my job and to be happy with my effort and outcomes, I would need to practice very differently than my colleagues.

Finding fulfillment within your vocation is achieved through balance. While I adhered to the medical group's metrics and goals, which prioritized high patient volumes, my goal was to treat every patient as if they were my only patient, as if they were my mother or father. Over the next several years, I carefully scrutinized and quietly modified the roles, responsibilities, and workflows for myself, the nurses, and our patients. Meanwhile, to ensure I met the medical group's performance targets, I simply worked longer hours. Therein was the ability to see more patients, while achieving my personal goals regarding patient experience and outcomes. In the end, perhaps not surprisingly, the changes the nurses, patients, and I made led to a thriving practice with lots of revenue for the medical group, a much more enjoyable and engaging work atmosphere for the staff and myself, and most importantly, a better experience and outcome for the patients. Other than a nagging discrepancy between how my peers and I practiced, I couldn't have been happier.

Following a decade of happiness and success in private practice, I accepted a healthcare executive role for the health system affiliated with my medical group. Specifically, I agreed to help doctors and nurses adapt to a very new and disruptive technology being deployed throughout U.S. hospitals and medical groups: the electronic health record (EHR). Over the next few years, I was responsible for assisting physicians with replacing their pens, paper charts, dictation recorders, and transcriptionists with computers, monitors, keyboards, and information technology (IT) staff.

From the beginning of this multiyear transition to a new EHR, it was quite evident that for most doctors across the United States, this transition was the single most traumatic event of their professional careers. Compounding this challenge was the reality that the newly deployed computerized medical record systems were expensive, poorly designed, had little to no ability to communicate with each other, and significantly eroded the time physicians and staff directly interacted with their patients and each other. As patients, both of my sisters navigated their healthcare systems utilizing EHRs while being treated for cancer and an autoimmune condition, no more informed or better cared for by the system that managed our mother's cancer treatment two decades earlier.

After working at the health system and repeatedly witnessing the traumatic impact of transitioning independent private practices onto the health system's EHR, it was evident that there were additional contributors to the staff's unhappiness. Following the acquisition of a private medical group by the health system, the newly employed physicians and the clinical staff were expected to follow new procedures and protocols that they did not quite understand or trust. Within weeks of becoming employees of a larger health organization, the doctors and the staff resigned themselves to help-lessly learning to use difficult tools and following questionable workflows with diminishing autonomy, mastery, and joy.

Sadly, my local experience reflected a larger national trend of the past decade inadvertently brought about by the implementation of EHRs by hospitals and medical groups. On a national level, the cost and complexity to implement, manage, and update these computer systems and the cor-responding workflows was so unexpectedly high and difficult that smaller private practices struggled to manage this transformation. Thus began a national wave of consolidation resulting in larger medical groups and health systems buying smaller private medical practices at an alarming rate. The cumulative disruption for hundreds of thousands of U.S. doctors over the past decade, in some ways, rivals the disruption we are all expe-riencing today due to the recent COVID-19 pandemic. The abrupt loss of familiar routines that served us so well has resulted in an alarming depth of pain and suffering. The less recognized and discussed consequence of rising unhappiness and dissatisfaction among physicians and clinical staff is the risk of worsening harm to patients.

After working as a healthcare executive, I can understand why so few happy and successful clinicians would consider replacing the daily gratifi-cation of caring for patients with the complex and difficult balancing act of leading large medical groups, hospitals, or health systems. Ironically, I won-der whether most physicians that historically gravitate to such leadership roles either did not enjoy direct patient care or weren't very good at it and therefore perhaps are even less well suited to be effective healthcare leaders. Thus, at times, it seems we are left with healthcare leaders who fail to rec-ognize or understand the broader consequences of marching forward with such disruptive strategies. While most healthcare executives are exposed to broad business and accounting concepts, few are specifically trained to effectively engage, manage, or influence physicians, nurses, or patients. Yet, at a minimum, being an effective healthcare leader requires an intimate understanding of practicing medicine, deeply caring about your constitu-ents, and possessing a sense of curiosity, courage, and humility. Whether in the past or present, encountering such gifted and talented leaders is disconcertingly infrequent, though I was fortunate to work with a few of them.

Over the past two decades, I have witnessed my profession transform from one of the most rewarding vocations to one reporting alarming statistics on physician unhappiness and dissatisfaction despite being in the top percent of U.S. earners. Even more frightening is the possibility that our focus and ability to ensure safe and effective care is also deteriorating. To some extent, our initial poor response to the COVID-19 pandemic hints at the underlying fragility of our current healthcare system. While everyone's commitment to providing excellent care is always unwavering, our ability to deliver on that promise continues to degrade at a staggering rate. Unless we seriously reevaluate and rethink our roles, responsibilities, workflows, and tools, we risk conforming to a flawed system and methodology despite most of us knowing better.

Today, I wonder whether I am misunderstanding reality because it seems so few of my peers or colleagues express similar concerns. Most continue to work as if the present model is the best we can do, while they benefit from a long tradition of respect and reward. Besides the rare article that reports almost unbelievable statistics on poor patient outcomes such as harm, death, and bankruptcy caused in part by our actions, there is only the rising level of unhappiness and dissatisfaction recently reported among physicians and nurses to suggest something is seriously wrong and needs to be addressed urgently.

As in the past, medicine's dilemma pervades all our lives. It remains difficult to recognize the insidious way in which we fail to care for our patients and each other. It is neither obvious how to solve these problems nor easy to challenge the status quo. Yet, if we do succeed, we can dramatically improve patient outcomes and clinical staff experience while lowering costs. Given all our collective experiences and shared hope for a safer, better healthcare experience, we are certainly capable of rethinking and redesigning who does what, where, how, when, and why.

If we continue the path of apathetic conformity, I predict we may soon have to more explicitly explain how we unintentionally, inadvertently, but consistently enable too many of our patients to be harmed. They or their families will ask us how we accepted such bad practices with so few safeguards. Why did we not speak out and do more to ensure their safety? How will we explain why we are failing to protect the very patients we took an oath to serve?

Over these pages, please see whether you can recognize the good and the bad of how medicine is practiced today.

Examining Medicine: How Do You Perceive the Practice of Medicine?

Step 1: Please answer the five questions below and score yourself at the end.

The Patient

Chris sat down with empty seats to either side of him. The few people nearby were evenly spaced apart, quietly awaiting their turn. Hopefully, today's annual visit wouldn't consume his entire afternoon like last year. A few weeks ago, while calling the doctor's office for a physical, he had remembered the nurse's advice and scheduled an early morning appointment. At his last visit, she had apologetically told him that was his best chance to get in and out quickly. More importantly, it meant that after seeing the doctor, he'd immediately go to the laboratory for his fasting bloodwork and then afterwards get a chance to grab an early lunch. So, while a bit hungry, overall, he was relaxed and ready. He pulled out his phone and waited for the doctor.

Which of the following is/are often true?
  A. When scheduling a routine visit with your doctor, normally you are given an appointment a few days or weeks from the time you called.
  B. Scheduling an appointment with your doctor in the early morning often results in less time spent at the doctor's office than an appointment scheduled in the afternoon, particularly if you have to get lab work done.
  C. For your annual physical exam visit, it is better for you to get your bloodwork completed a few days before the appointment rather than after you have seen your doctor.

D. Two of the above

E. All of the above

THE MEDICAL ASSISTANT / NURSE

The morning was going well. Today, traffic had been light, so Maria made it to work in under an hour. That gave her enough time to clear her fax folder, scan the row of test results posted on her electronic health record (EHR) inbox, and listen to the overnight voicemails, all before checking in the first patient of the morning. Fortunately, the voicemails had delivered a bit of good news. The last two patients for today had canceled, so she had a chance to get home on time as long as no one added any more patients. She even began to wonder whether she may get a chance to eat lunch at the cafeteria rather than sneaking it in at her desk while juggling patients and the steady stream of incoming EHR tasks that flooded her inbox all day long. She glanced at the name of the first patient of the morning before walking out to the waiting room and calling out for "Chris T.?"

Which of the following is/are often true?

A. For most doctor offices, the medical assistant is expected to check in patients, check voicemails, check faxes, and execute orders/tasks from the doctor.

B. For most doctor offices, approving an appointment for a sick patient to be seen the same day usually requires the approval of the doctor and/or their nurse.

C. Clinical staff are rarely incentivized or rewarded to see more patients per day.

D. Two of the above

E. All of the above

THE DOCTOR

Joanna walked outside and crossed the street to her medical office, enjoying the brisk morning air and the hot coffee she had collected from the doctor's lounge at the hospital. Luckily, she was a few minutes ahead of schedule because both of her hospitalized patients were located on the same floor, and more importantly, both were getting better. One patient may even go home tomorrow if the social worker could work it out with the family and the home health agency.

After entering through the side door of the clinic, she walked by the charging station to remove her laptop and bring it to her cubicle. As she waited to access her EHR, she sorted through the paperwork on her desk, initially focusing on the yellow sticky notes she had made as important reminders. If all went well, she'd have enough time to review today's patient test results and fire off the corresponding electronic tasks to her staff before stepping into the examination room to see her first patient.

Twenty minutes later, she stood in front of the closed door to the patient room, balancing her laptop in her arm as she scanned through the patient's EHR. She noted he was here for his annual exam and otherwise doing well. A quick and easy start to the day, only distracted by the nagging fact that her bad diabetic patient had once again broken his promise to follow up and instead canceled his appointment at the end of the day. She didn't recognize the name of the other cancelation but wondered whether the staff would fill these two open slots with some other patients or, perhaps if she were lucky, she may get to use the extra time to finish her clinic notes at the office rather than later tonight in bed.

She opened the door and greeted Chris with a warm smile.

Which of the following is/are often true?

A. Most doctors try to see their hospital patients in the morning before they start seeing their clinic patients.

B. On most days, doctors would prefer to go home earlier to see their families rather than see more patients.

C. On most days, physicians spend more hours documenting their clinic notes, managing telephone messages, and performing other administrative tasks rather than directly speaking and caring for their patients.

D. Two of the above

E. All of the above

THE ADMINISTRATOR

Despite serving as the medical group's administrator for the past four years, Peter still braced himself for the monthly executive committee meetings with the five physician leaders of the group. He carefully reviewed the spreadsheet one last time, confirming the stubborn fact that the number of same-day patient cancelations continued to exceed the same-day requests for appointments by patients despite their latest attempt to centralize scheduling. Otherwise, the end-of-the-quarter numbers looked good, so he closed his laptop and quickly prepared to walk upstairs to ensure everything was in order for the start of today's meeting.

As he hustled up the stairs, he remembered how last year, the executive committee had agreed to invest in launching virtual video visits with some of the younger, more willing physicians. Unfortunately, they didn't release funding until a few months ago, when the pandemic struck and suddenly it wasn't an option. Luckily, he had been able to purchase enough laptops with extra batteries, secure the proper teleconferencing licenses, and redesign the waiting areas and staff areas. Crazy days and nights went on for weeks, but he and his team set up the doctors to conduct virtual patient visits. He marveled at how decisive the leadership could be in a crisis and how supportive and responsive the entire staff was to the radical changes in their schedules, workflows, and responsibilities.

While the revenue loss from the reduced office visits was mostly offset with the widespread adoption of video and telephone visits, he worried about the future. If more visits continued to be done virtually then would they need less clinical staff in the office? Perhaps they may require more ancillary staff to help clean the patient rooms between visits? Would it be better to transition the shared cubicles back into private offices that a few of the more senior physicians retained?

Despite these concerns and the fatigue of working ten- to twelve-hour days for the past few months, he was also quietly excited about today's meeting. Last month's elections had resulted in two younger physicians being voted on to the executive committee. Perhaps because, for the first time ever, there were now two working moms on the committee, Peter felt some long-debated policies regarding improving same-day patient appointments, flexible staff work hours, and job sharing could be tried and tested. Perhaps . . .

As he reached the conference room, he tucked away these swirling possibilities and immediately noticed that one of his favorite physicians, Dr. Joanna Casey, a newly elected committee member, was already hunched over her laptop munching on a sandwich while pecking at the keyboard with her free hand. Soon all the executive committee physicians would arrive and the entire flock would be eating, pecking, and listening as Peter ran through the agenda. He silenced his phone, took a deep breath, and waited.

Which of the following is/are often true?
   A. Overall, in the medical profession, while male doctors outnumber female doctors nearly 2:1, in 2019, for the first time ever the majority of U.S. medical students were women.
   B. Most private practice medical groups are led by a few senior physicians who continue to see patients while working with their administrator to manage the business side of the practice.
   C. Under the pressure of time, doctors and clinical staff frequently multitask, which may lead to errors and even harm to patients.
   D. Two of the above
   E. All of the above

THE FAMILY

Judy was still on hold as she waited at the traffic light. She had to get to the pharmacy to pick up her mom's blood pressure medication before they closed, and she was getting frustrated. It was always difficult to speak with her mom's doctor or her nurse, but over the years, she had learned it was better to wait and speak with someone than leave a voicemail.

Finally, the nurse answered and apologized for the delay. Judy carefully explained the situation—last week, she had taken her mom to see the doctor, had lab work done, and they were told to keep her mom on the same medications. Then earlier today, a voicemail from the pharmacy told them to come in and pick up their blood pressure medication. So what should she do? Was everything okay with her mom's lab tests, as they hadn't heard anything from the doctor's office?

After listening to Judy, the nurse placed her on hold again.

As Judy drove to the pharmacy, she remembered what her friend at work had told her about getting her mom set up on a mail order medication refill service. Her friend loved it because they automatically shipped a ninety-day supply of her medications directly to the house. And it was cheaper. While Judy would love to avoid having to drive to the pharmacy once or twice every month, she suspected it wouldn't work for her mother because the doctors were always adjusting her medications. Still, it was worth asking the doctor about it because it might save them some money as well as time.

The nurse's voice came back on the phone and she explained that the doctor had lowered the dose of one of her mom's blood pressure medications after her mom's lab tests noted her potassium level was a bit lower than she liked. The doctor had sent an electronic order with the new dose to the pharmacy, who notified the patient. The nurse reassured Judy that they were continuing the same medication but just at half the dose. The doctor felt this would prevent the problem from happening again, though they planned to check her potassium level at the next office visit in two months.

Judy understood and thanked the nurse. Then she asked the nurse whether they could cut her mom's current blood pressure medication in half with their pill splitter. The nurse paused and said, "I think so, but just check to make sure the tablet is scored, that it has a groove in the middle," and then hung up.

Judy pulled into the pharmacy parking lot and tried to think what else she needed to buy for the house while she was here.

Which of the following is/are often true?
- A. If a test result is abnormal, your doctor's office will try to let you know.
- B. When refilling medication requests, your doctor's staff tries to make sure the correct medication name, dosage, and frequency are being refilled but they usually *do not check* to ensure the necessary labs have been done recently or if there are any potentially harmful drug interactions with any of your other medications.
- C. Each year, more than 250,000 patients die due to medical errors, which makes it the third leading cause of death in the United States.
- D. Two of the above
- E. All of the above

Step II: Score Calculation
Please score your exam by totaling the number of points using the following scale:
  1 point for each A
  2 points for each B
  3 points for each C
  4 points for each D
  5 points for each E

Step III: Total score and your results
    5–8 Grateful for our approach to healthcare
    9–12 Satisfied with our approach to healthcare
    13–16 Concerned with our approach to healthcare
    17–20 Frustrated with our approach to healthcare
    21–25 Afraid of our approach to healthcare

Physicians and their teams along with patients and their families are meant to work together, each contributing their effort and expertise working towards the common goal of better health and understanding. Your answers to these questions may reveal whether you believe our healthcare delivery system is dutifully safeguarding her citizens and living up to this promise or we are falling short and inadvertently harming our patients and clinical staff. Depending on your answers, our paths may cross again as we each do our part to make healthcare safer and better for all.

Par Bolina, M.D.
Internal Medicine

Acknowledgments

I owe a debt of gratitude to countless authors who introduced me to so many remarkable characters who served as teachers, mentors, and role models. Over a lifetime of reading books and stories, these characters influenced my purpose, values, and decision making. Alongside my parents, the characters in those books are my most reliable source of inspiration and courage.

I am deeply grateful to the original ninety contributors of *Becoming Doctors* and especially grateful to the twenty-four contributors of this book. Among this group, Dr. Sue Rhee has our collective gratitude for creating such a wonderful cover illustration reflecting our aspirations and struggles as physicians. Equally critical to the success of this endeavor was the immeasurable contribution of Angie Wilson. As in most success stories, a chance meeting plus a sense of adventure accompanied by courage, trust, effort, and perseverance led to our collaboration and friendship without which this sequel anthology would not have been possible. I also wish to thank Larry Carpenter and Shane Crabtree and the entire team at Clovercroft Publishing for their valuable guidance. Finally, I wish to thank my sisters and closest friends for their support and encouragement on these two journeys.

My hope is that these words capture the depth of my gratitude for those mentioned and to the many more left unmentioned. Whether new or old, friendship is a powerful force that enables wonderful outcomes.

Par Bolina

ABOUT THE EDITOR

Par Bolina, born in London in 1970, relocated to Chicago in 1979. He later graduated from the University of Illinois at Chicago College of Medicine in 1996. During his time in medical school, he edited and published *Becoming Doctors*, an anthology written by ninety-one medical students from over fifty medical schools across the United States. After completing his residency training in Massachusetts, he relocated to Nashville, Tennessee, to work as an internist. By 2010, his interest in improving patient and clinician experience initially led him to become a chief medical informatics officer at one of the nation's largest nonprofit health systems and later as chief innovation officer in the private sector. Presently, he continues to develop new methods and workflows for clinicians and patients to deliver and receive better, safer care.